Trauma of the Middle Ear

Advances in
Oto-Rhino-Laryngology

Vol. 35

Series Editor
C. R. Pfaltz, Basel

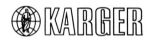

Basel · München · Paris · London · New York · New Delhi · Singapore · Tokyo · Sydney

Trauma of the Middle Ear

Clinical Findings, Postmortem Observations and Results of Experimental Studies

Michael Strohm
Department of Otorhinolaryngology, University of Tübingen,
Tübingen, FRG

14 figures and 86 tables, 1986

Translated from the German by *Jürgen Tonndorf*

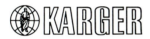

Basel · München · Paris · London · New York · New Delhi · Singapore · Tokyo · Sydney

Advances in Oto-Rhino-Laryngology

National Library of Medicine, Cataloging in Publication
    Strohm, Michael.
    Trauma of the middle ear: clinical findings, postmortem observations, and results of experimental
    studies /
    Michael Strohm. — Basel; New York, Karger, 1986. —
    (Advances in oto-rhino-laryngology; vol. 35)
    Bibliography: p.
    Includes index.
    1. Ear, Middle — injuries II. Title III. Series
    W1 AD701 v. 35 [WV230 S921t]
    ISBN 3-8055-4087-6

Drug Dosage
    The author and publisher have exerted every effort to ensure that drug selection and dosage set
    forth in this text are in accord with current recommendations and practice at the time of
    publication. However, in view of ongoing research, changes in government regulations, and the
    constant flow of information relating to drug therapy and drug reactions, the reader is urged to
    check the package insert for each drug for any change in indications and dosage and for added
    warnings and precautions. This is particularly important when the recommended agent is a new
    and/or infrequently employed drug.

Contents

Acknowledgements

To Prof. Dr. *D. Plester*, head of the ENT-Department of the University of Tübingen, I wish to express my heartfelt gratitude for stimulating my interest in microsurgery of the traumatized ear. I am grateful for his continuous support and interest and for enabling me to do this investigation. To Prof. *Bohle* (head of the Pathologic Institute of the University of Tübingen) and to Prof. *Mallach* (head of the Institute of Forensic Medicine of the University of Tübingen), my sincere thanks for allowing me to examine the postmortem specimens. My colleagues Prof. *Steinbach* and Dr. *Heumann* helped in performing the animal experiments and the histological examinations, to them, I also express my gratitude.

I especially want to thank Prof. *Tonndorf* (New York), who not only translated this paper, but also reviewed it critically and who gave me helpful advice.

Finally I appreciate the excellent counseling and cooperation provided by the editor, Prof. *Pfaltz*, and the staff of the S. Karger AG throughout the printing and publication process.

M. Strohm

Foreword

Growing industrialization and the increasing number of traffic accidents often lead to middle ear trauma at different sites and of varying severity. Special problems of partial or sometimes complete destruction of the temporal bone have frequently — and often controversially — been discussed in the otological literature.

In the present book, Dr. *Strohm* describes the findings, microsurgical techniques and results in more than 800 such cases treated for middle ear trauma during the last 13 years at the ENT Clinic at Tübingen University. These cases include immediate and delay surgery (sometimes decades after the trauma) as well as facial nerve trauma and posttraumatic cholesteatoma. Early or late surgery for eardrum perforation, the reconstruction of the ossicular chain and the leakage of CSF after fracture of the base of the skull are also discussed in detail. The corrective procedures described by Dr. *Strohm* are presented clearly and the rationale behind these procedures is argued convincingly.

The chapter on trauma of the round window or its membrane might be of special interest nowadays, especially since the diagnosis 'rupture of the round window membrane' is made frequently but, in our experience, far too often.

This book provides in one comprehensive volume the principles of modern ear surgery after trauma in the era of tympanoplasty. It covers the experience gained in a great number of patients and should prove very useful to postgraduate students and to every otolaryngologist dealing with surgery of the middle ear and the skull base.

D. Plester

1. Introduction

Historically, the traumatology of the middle ear (ME) was developed in four separate phases, each of them characterized by a different attitude on the part of the otologists as regards lesions of the ME system.

During the second half of the 19th century, the first phase, basic knowledge was accumulated about the origin of skull-base fractures and their underlying mechanisms. Most of it was contributed by surgeons: simple skull fractures were differentiated from depressed fractures [294, 452]. The modes of origin of longitudinal and transverse fractures of the temporal bone (TB) and their characteristic appearances were also assessed [190, 452].

During the second phase, around the turn of the century, traumatic lesions of middle and inner ears were correlated with fractures of the skull base [20, 266]. In 1906 already, *Zalewski* [473] studied the resistance of the tympanic membrane (TM) to differences in air pressure across it; but his results did not find immediate clinical applications. The book *Die Verletzungen des Ohres* (Trauma of the Ear) by *Passow* [339] gave a comprehensive, and impressive, summary on the state-of-the-art with respect to the etiology and symptomatology of such lesions. The concepts presented appear almost modern.

Postmortem studies [443] performed on TB obtained from persons who had died following skull traumata, as well as clinical findings [267, 449, 450] led to direct surgical interventions during the third phase. Such interventions were recommended especially in those cases in which the trauma had created an open communication between the endocranium and the pneumatized mastoid spaces, constituting a life-threatening complication, real or potential. *Voss* [449, 450] therefore separated curative surgery from preventive surgery, depending on whether an otogenic intracranial infection was already present or merely imminent. The aim of the surgical intervention was the permanent eradication of infection. However, no attention was paid to the maintenance and/or restoration of the ME and its function.

Beginning in the 1950s, the concept of tympanoplasty, i.e. the preservation of function and/or its restoration by means of microsurgery of *infected* ears, was extended to the care of *traumatized* ears. This represents the fourth phase. The introduction of the sulfonamides and the antibiotics had lessened the need for curative, and especially for preventive, surgery. Hence, microsurgical reconstruction of the ME gained in importance. *Escher*, in his 1964 monograph, entitled *Funktionelle Ohrchirurgie traumatischer Mittelohrläsionen* (Reconstructive Surgery of Traumatic Middle Ear Lesions), reviewed this topic in quite some detail. In particular he wrote: 'Such lesions are much more varied than heretofore realized; and the repair of defective middle ears may lead to considerable functional improvements. Systematic surgical interventions permit to recognize incipient destructive lesions, such as ossicular osteitis and the ingrowth of keratinizing epithelium into the middle ear, and permit their repair.'

In 1964, *Escher* [99] was still of the opinion that surgical intervention had to be postponed until the direct sequelae of the trauma had a chance to subside. More recent authors, however, demanded early surgery. *Armstrong* [13], for example, warned against this form of 'watchful neglect'. He wrote: 'Facial lacerations are carefully approximated with fine sutures to achieve a pleasing cosmetic result, but too often the tympanic membrane receives little attention... This is regrettable because it places cosmetic appearances above functional results. This double standard is encouraged by our cosmetically orientated society, that is, if it doesn't show, it doesn't matter'. This statement that originally concerned only traumatic ruptures of the TM is even more important with regard to perilymphatic fistulae and posttraumatic facial nerve (FN) palsies. The demand for early otosurgical intervention represents the most important progress in the field of surgical repair of traumatic ME lesions in the last 10 years. It was demanded that every patient, who suffered an ME trauma, should be seen by an otologist with training in ME surgery. This otologist had to make the decision whether immediate intervention is indicated or whether a wait-and-see attitude may be warranted.

In an effort to provide a rationale for early intervention, the patient records of the ENT Department at Tübingen University, FRG, were systematically scrutinized with particular reference to trauma of the ear and its sequelae. At this institution, microsurgery of the ear is being conducted according to quite uniform therapeutic standards. Also assessed was the diagnostic value of roentgenological examination of patients with such lesions. Postmortem studies on TM obtained from persons who had died from their injuries served to demonstrate the structural changes induced by the trauma. Lastly, experiments were conducted on lesions of the TM and those of the round window (RW) membrane and their self-repair.

2. Materials and Methods

All statements made in the present monograph concerning ME trauma are based on the evaluation of clinical observations, postmortem findings and roentgenograms; the latter are important with regard to the following two types of trauma: (1) TM lesions and (2) TB fractures, especially when they include FN injuries. For these reasons the methods of examination of all types of injuries are reported together. On the other hand, each experimental study had one specific aim; their special methodology is therefore described separately in each appropriate chapter.

2.1. Clinical Examinations

Records of all patients treated for traumatic lesions of the ear during the time period from 1968 to 1980 inclusively were culled from the departmental archives and from the operating-room repository. From each patient's record, the following information, if available, was extracted: (1) past history; (2) findings on admission, including pure-tone audiograms and X-ray pictures; (3) reports on clinical management and/or surgical interventions, and (4) clinical findings and the final audiogram at the time of discharge. The entire information could not be collected in every case. For example, the past history of patients seen only in the clinic on referral from other departments was no longer available, since it had only been given on the referral slip. Furthermore, audiological and X-ray examinations had, in many cases, already been performed by the referring physician; hence, there was no appropriate record in the departmental archives. Lastly, some patients did not present themselves for the final examination.

Some patients were included in the present study even when their records were incomplete. The reports and findings that were available served to answer some questions, e.g. about the frequency of the various causes of different lesions or about their location.

The present study comprises a total of 691 patients; 463 of them had undergone surgery and 228 had been treated by conservative means. During the report period, otosurgery was carried out on a grand total of approximately 20,000 patients. This means that 2.3 % of all surgical interventions on the ear were carried out on account of traumatic lesions.

2.2. Postmortem Observations

During the years 1978–80, all temporal bones were removed whenever a head post was performed in the case of a fatal skull-brain trauma. The autopsies were conducted either at the Institute of Forensic Medicine or at that of Pathology of Tübingen University. There was a total of 46 cases. Of them, 43 represented blunt skull traumata and the remaining 3 gunshot injuries. After exclusion of all material damaged during autopsy, 89 temporal bones remained for detailed examination. After fixation in formalin, the lining of the external ear canal (EEC), the TM and the course of fracture lines, if present, were examined under the operating microscope. Still under microscopic control, the soft tissues were removed from the mastoid and from the basal surface of each bone. With the aid of a surgical drill, the floor of the hypotympanum was opened from the tubal ostium all the way to the stylomastoid foramen. Removal of adjacent portions of the floor of the EEC made it possible to deflect the lower part of the TM, enabling the experimenter to inspect a large part of the ME space, including the RW niche. Fracture lines were followed by taking down the mastoid. Findings made during the course of these preparations were documented either by drawings or by photography.

2.3. Roentgenological Findings

For many patients, X-ray pictures were available in the projections of *Schüller* and/or *Stenvers*. For some patients, lateral-skull X-ray pictures also existed. All pictures were evaluated from two aspects: (1) the degree of pneumatization and (2) the diagnosis of fractures.

2.3.1. Assessment of Pneumatization

It was of interest to learn if different types of TM lesions as well as the course of their repair could be correlated with the degree of mastoid pneumatization. *Diamant* [71] demonstrated a correlation coefficient of 0.94 ± 0.14 between the projected area of the air spaces as seen in lateral skull X-rays with their extension into the pyramidal apex. *Flisberg and Zsigmond* [125] compared planimetric and volumetric measurements of the mastoid air cells; they found a similar correlation coefficient, i.e. 0.88 in normal, healthy ears. These two findings indicate that planimetric assessments of the projected areas of the 3-dimensional pneumatic air spaces on Schüller X-ray pictures render a relative, but meaningful, measure of the degree of pneumatization, although they do not give absolute volumes. This information is quite sufficient with respect to the present question, i.e. for comparing the degree of pneumatization with the vulnerability of the TM and its tendency to heal.

There are two potential sources of error in the planimetric evaluation of Schüller X-ray pictures:

(1) They are not teleprojections, i.e. the object is not projected in its true size; rather, they are divergent projections, i.e. the projected picture is larger than the object. Nevertheless, if the same, identical equipment is used throughout the series, the magnification should remain about constant. For the equipment used in our department, the range of variation was calculated. It amounted to approximately $\pm 0.25\%$. Suffice it to say, however, that neither the magnification nor its range of variation are of any significance, as long as one is only interested in the *relative* extent of pneumatization.

(2) The direction of the projection may vary slightly from one patient to another since it is determined by a number of landmarks on the skull that may differ in different patients. Somewhat schematically, one may regard the air spaces as forming a pyramid with its base parallel to the lateral surface of the mastoid. Since the center of the X-ray beam does not always coincide with the axis of the pyramid, the projection of its base (which yields the

desired measure of the degree of pneumatization) might be distorted. Calculations indicated that the resulting error was not larger than approximately ± 0.28%.

These two considerations demonstrate that the planimetric evaluation of routine Schüller roentgenograms renders an index number that is sufficiently accurate for the purpose at hand, i.e. to indicate the relative volume of the mastoid air spaces.

2.3.2. Diagnosis of Fractures

It was of further interest to learn if and to what degree of confidence the existence of a fracture line could be established and its course determined on the basis of routine, clinical X-ray pictures. In contrast to the planimetric assessment of mastoid pneumatization there was no other objective method available for the verification of suspected fracture lines. Hence, the possibility existed that the evaluation of the X-ray pictures might be influenced, even in a subconscious manner, by other clinical details known to the reviewer. To avoid this potential pitfall, the evaluation was done in a blind-study fashion: A medical student collated all clinical and surgical records of patients with skull traumata, for whom X-ray pictures were available. He then forwarded nothing but the roentgenograms to the author for their evaluation. Finally, drawings made of the X-ray findings were correlated with the clinical records.

Note. Results obtained by various authors will be quoted in the chapters discussing the resistance of the TM and of the RW membrane to differential pressures across them, as well as in those chapters describing the general effects of barotrauma. For proper comparison of the different results obtained from the literature, the following relations were used:

$$1 \text{ bar} = 1,000 \text{ mbar} = 1.019 \text{ at}$$
$$= 760 \text{ mm Hg} = 750 \text{ Torr} = 14.5 \text{ psi}$$
$$= 10^6 \text{ dyn/cm}^2 = 100 \text{ N/cm}^2 = 100 \text{ kPa}.$$

For example, 180 dB SPL are aproximately equivalent to an absolute pressure of 2×10^5 dyn/cm^2; and 200 dB SPL to an absolute pressure of 2×10^6 dyn/cm^2 = 2 at.

3. Tympanic Membrane Lesions

Strictly speaking, EEC injuries should not be included under the heading of *Trauma to the Middle Ear*. Their descriptions are therefore omitted from the present monograph. Admittedly, EEC lesions often extend into the ME (e.g. a cholesteatoma behind an EEC stenosis; fractures of the EEC walls as part of a longitudinal TB fracture). These lesions will be handled in the appropriate chapters on ME pathology.

The discussion of ME lesions must logically start with those of the TM, its most accessible part.

3.1. Etiology

Injuries via the EEC can directly affect the TM. They may be mechanical or thermal in nature; or they might have been produced by an air pressure differential across the membrane, brought about by changes in atmospheric pressure that are not compensated by identical changes in ME pressure. Furthermore, TM lesions may result from transient osseous deformations produced by a blunt skull trauma. *Passow* [339], after a perusal of the pertinent literature, gave the relative incidence of TM lesions as 0.43–2.16% of all disorders of the ear. His higher number agrees well with that of the Tübingen ENT Department (2.3%; cf. chapter 2.1 above).

3.1.1. Lesions of Mechanical Origin

As is well known, attempts to clean the EEC are the most frequent causes of mechanically induced TM injuries. The instruments used for that purpose include cotton applicators and others that are even less suitable, such as hair pins, rat-tail combs, matches, etc. [75, 357, 397, 459]. Long, slender particles of matter, such as twigs or pieces of straw, may accidentally enter the EEC and perforate the TM [51, 75, 339]. Since the EEC is slightly S-shaped, the *posterosuperior* quadrant of the TM lies directly in the projection of the canal axis. Theoretically at least, this portion of the TM should be especially vulnerable. A number of authors [13, 51, 81, 287] called attention to this fact, mentioning the potential danger to the ME structures behind it. *Zaufal* [475–477] and *Passow* [339], however, found that lesions produced mechanically via the EEC are more frequently located in the *anteroinferior* quadrant. After conducting experiments in cadaver ears, they concluded that instruments introduced into the EEC are reflected by the posterior wall in a generally anteroinferior direction. It was only after pushing the tragus anteriorly that they were able to perforate the posterior portion of the TM.

In addition to sharp tools that may perforate the TM directly, small foreign bodies are capable of doing the same, such as pieces of cerumen, cotton plugs, insects and various things children put into the EEC during play (pebbles, beans, buds of pussy willows, etc.). A foreign body wedged into the EEC, especially when it is liable to swell up, may cause an infectious edema, involve the TM, and lead to a suppurative otitis media and even to a mastoiditis [313]. *Chalier and Rousset* [cited after 313] described the case of a child, 3 years of age, who died from tetanus contracted after a pebble had been put into his EEC. Earlier, *Kiesselbach* [239] had collected 13 similar cases from the literature; foreign bodies lodged in the EEC had been the causes of death in all of them.

Often, it is not the foreign body that ruptures the TM directly, but rather misguided attempts to remove it. Into this category belong manipulations in the EEC of a frightened child that cries and fights the physician [397], and also attempts to remove a foreign body by means of a forceps. Frequently, such attempts succeed only in pushing the material deeper and deeper into the EEC and finally through the TM into the ME [221].

Laceration of the TM during the course of a successful extraction is probably a rare event. *Mosher* [313] described the extraction of a tick, the head of which was so deeply buried in the TM that a piece of it was torn out during the removal of the arthropode.

Finally, although it is certainly the method of choice for cleaning the EEC, even irrigating it may occasionally lacerate the TM, especially when the canula is accidentally pushed too deeply into the EEC [99]. Strictly speaking, such TM lesions are not really caused by the foreign object itself; rather, they are iatrogenic in nature.

3.1.2. Lesions of Thermal Origin

A foreign body intruding into the EEC, without touching the walls, should not be expected to possess sufficient kinetic energy to directly penetrate the TM. Nevertheless, serious injuries are produced by hot particles, such as arcs from a grindstone, or red-glowing pieces of metal or cinder entering the EEC during welding or steel-pouring operations. The first description of a TM lesion produced in this manner was given by *Alexander* [3]. While steel was being poured, a drop of liquid metal was flung into the left EEC of the patient, immediately making him unconscious. Later on, he suffered from dizziness, and the ear in question became deaf; there was fetid discharge and a facial palsy. Since no lesions could be seen in the EEC, the patient's account met initially with skepticism. Surgery, however, uncovered a grain-sized piece of metal lying in the hypotympanum.

Papers published later (3 cases [165]; 1 case [275]) reported TM burns that had left the EEC completely untouched. *Güttich* [165] thought that some protection might be provided by the ceruminal lining of the canal walls. His other notion, i.e. that this might be due to the ballistic curve of the object flying through an EEC that is likewise curved, appears to be rather farfetched.

Heermann [186] culled 15 cases of TM or ME burns respectively from the records of the Krupp Hospital, Essen, FRG. All of these injuries had been incurred during ore-smelting or metal-pouring operations. The author was able to demonstrate that the seriousness of the injury was correlated with the size of the foreign body (i.e. probably with its thermal capacity). The absolute temperatures are invariably so high — 1,200°C during welding operations [304] — that small individual differences do not appear to play a role.

Several, more extensive series were published later (11 cases [133]; 8 cases [288]; 13 cases [313]; 44 cases [371]; 32 cases [446]). All of their authors reported essentially the same findings: as a rule, the left ear was involved (although the right ear in left-handers). The perforation was usually located in the anteroinferior quadrant. In the case of very small foreign bodies, the perforation did not become visible until a few days had elapsed following the original injury [371, 446]. Cerumen, if present, protected the ear canal by slowing down the speed of the intruding object [371, 446]. *Mosher* [313] expressed the opinion that a strong serous discharge from the ear might dislodge a foreign body. *Schein* [371] never detected a foreign body in the ME. *Heermann* [186], however, had to remove one each from the ME of 2 of his patients. In some cases, the inner ear was also found to be involved [186, 288, 446]. *Heermann* [186] furthermore saw an FN disruption caused by a piece of hot metal and also a posttraumatic meningitis that led to the death of the patient.

Scalding of the TM by hot liquids appears to occur only rarely. The first such case was reported by *Wederstrandt* [457]; its cause was molten lead. *Walb* [453] also described such an injury; it was produced by steam. Scalding by hot water [258, 288], by hot oil [411] and by a hot plastic [364] was also reported. In the last case, a rather severe inner-ear impairment was observed.

3.1.3. Lesions Caused by Air-Pressure Differences across the Tympanic Membrane

The resistance of the TM against an air pressure differential on its two sides was first studied experimentally by *Schmidekam* [373]. He employed membranes preserved in alcohol. Ruptures occurred when the air pressure differential exceeded 1,430 or 1,680 mm Hg, respectively. *Gruber* [155] applied compressed air to TM obtained from fresh human cadavers, but failed to rupture them. *Zalewski* [473], as was already mentioned, was the first to conduct systematic experiments of this kind. Later experimenters were unable to add any more details to his original findings or to exceed his series of 232 temporal bones. (Aberrant results — i.e. maximal pressures: 6 atm [305], 0.5 atm [261] — do not appear sufficiently documented.) Therefore, *Zalewski's* results are still valid today:

(1) 66% of all normal, healthy TM ruptured at a differential air pressure between 1 and 2 atm (760 and 1,520 mm Hg (median value: 1,209 mm Hg; minimal value: 280 mm Hg; maximal value: 2,080 mm Hg). (Corresponding values reported by *Keller* [231]: median value: 1,292 mm Hg; extreme values: 724 and 1,706 mm Hg, respectively.)

(2) Ruptures were invariably located in pars tensa, as a rule in its anteroinferior quadrant. When scars were present, it was usually there that the TM had yielded.

(3) Almost invariably, ruptures were singular, either in the form of radially directed slits or of triangles with their bases facing the annulus. The fibrous annulus itself or the region of the umbo were never involved. (The latter observation agrees with the electron microscopic findings of *Graham* [485], who demonstrated that the umbo is enmeshed in a dense fibrous network belonging to the membrana propria.)

(4) As the rule, the edges of the perforations were folded-in at the middle ear side. The sudden pressure release had occasionally thrown pieces of epidermis or of cerumen into the ME.

Zalewski [473] as well as most other, later experimenters applied only quasistatic pressure changes. The question was repeatedly raised if the TM might react differently when exposed to a dynamically changing pressure pulse [232, 423]. Only *Keller* [231] attempted to answer this question. He found no difference in the resistance of the TM of cadaver ears when exposed to air pressures that changed either slowly or relatively fast. (This is a surprising and quite unexplained finding.)

In live persons also, the pressure differential may either rise slowly — its effects are usually described under the heading of barotrauma — or there may be a fast-rising, almost explosive, pressure pulse — its effect is called a blast injury or 'pressure wave trauma' [105].

The most widely known and most frequent causes of barotrauma are changes in altitude during airplane flights or changes in depth during diving. The effects on the ear that occur during airplane flights were studied mainly during World War Two (WW II) [e.g. 279]. Diving accidents involving the ear were described in a number of papers published mainly in the USA and in Australia [53, 108, 130, 261].

Under either condition, the causes of the ear injuries are easily understood: any increment in depth by 10 m in (incompressible) water raises the environmental pressure by 1 atm (760 mm Hg). In (compressible) air, however, the density decreases with increasing altitude; therefore, the relation is nonlinear, i.e. the altitude increments that produce given changes in environmental air pressure become the larger the higher the reference altitude. Numerically, air pressure p for altitude h is given by the exponential equation [196]:

$$p = p_0 e^{-\frac{h}{7992\,m}}$$

where p_0 = reference pressure, normally 1 atm = 760 mm Hg.

This equation indicates that, in gross approximation, at altitudes between zero and 3,000 m above sea level altitude *in*crements of 100 m correspond approximately to pressure *de*crements of 9.2 mm Hg [279].

Ascent in air as well as ascent under water decreases the environmental pressure acting in the EEC while the ME pressure stays (initially) unchanged. This produces a pressure differential across the TM, the lower pressure being on the outside. Whenever the intratympanic pressure exceeds that in the nasopharynx by 15 — 20 mm Hg, the Eustachian tube is passively forced open, the excess air being literally spilled from the ME [176, 211, 279, 319, 344]. The ME usually retains only a small amount of positive pressure, i.e. about 3–6 mm Hg [279]. The latter value of course varies from one individual to another. In the extreme case, the tube may stay permanently open, making relative pressure increases in the ME impossible.

The above autoregulatory mechanism fails to act when only the pressure in the EEC is lowered, but that in the nasopharynx remains unaltered. Detailed studies on this subject were conducted by *Ingelstedt and Örtegren* [210]. A report by *McCracken* [278] represents a case in point: a girl explored the ear canal of her boyfriend with her tongue. When she suddenly withdrew the tongue, the pressure in the external canal was lowered to such an extent that the TM was ruptured.

The nasopharyngeal pressure is also maintained, while that one in the EEC is decreasing, when an *untrained* diver refrains from exhaling during his ascent. TM are frequently ruptured in this manner during diving-school exercises. *Trained* divers, on the other hand, open their tubes so easily and without any apparent effort that they themselves are hardly aware of it [494].

The tubal mechanism responsible for its passive opening apparently becomes impaired during general anesthesia. *Owens* et al. [334] reported that the diffusion of nitrous oxygen into the ME creates a positive pressure. In 2 cases, this ultimately led to TM ruptures, but the TM in question had shown scars due to earlier disease processes. (Other things being equal, equilibration of a positive pressure in the ME is easier than that of a negative pressure for reasons that will become clear presently.)

Diffusion of N_2O into body cavities is known to produce positive pressures. This diffusion is more pronounced than the (simultaneous) discharge of N_2. While the ratios of the coefficients of *solution* of N_2 and of N_2O in the blood are 1:34, those of *diffusion* are 1:29.7. The maximal positive presssure that could be produced in this manner was calculated; it amounts to 34.2 mm Hg [341].

An excess air pressure in the ME may also cause TM lesions, but this occurs only rarely because the ME orifice of the Eustachian tube is a rigid osseous funnel that usually does not impair the discharge of air. Occasionally, however, when untrained divers undergo large pressure changes several times and rapidly in succession, the repeated insults produce an edema of the ME mucosa. If the ME pressure is once more elevated, it presses the (loose) edematous mucosa tightly into the tubal opening, thus preventing equilibration. There is acute pain and the TM is bulging, but hardly injected. If politzerization does not help, a small stab incision of the TM is required. There is prompt relief and the incision heals in a day or two [494].

More frequently, the cause of ME lesions lies in a relative *reduction* of ME pressure, i.e. in a relative *increase* of pressure in the external canal. However, the air needed for pressure equilibration cannot be brought passively from the nasopharynx into the ME via the Eustachian tube. Its nasopharyngeal torus is quite soft and is compressed under the effect of an increased external air pressure. An active opening is required, which can be produced by swallowing, yawning, execution of the Valsalva maneuver, and similar measures.

This mechanism may be impaired: (1) by nasopharyngeal infections, septal deviations, adenoidal hyperplasia [62, 240, 242, 279]; (2) by a decrease in surfactants in the tubal mucus [47, 124], and (3) when, once more in untrained persons, the descent occurs so fast that there is no time for forcing the tube open. When the pressure differential thus produced exceeds 60–80 mm Hg, the external pressure acting on the soft torus tubarius prevents the tube from being forced open [70, 124, 241, 272, 279]. In that case, the TM is exposed to the full differential pressure and so is the ME mucosa. Consequently, whenever the pressure differential exceeds 300 mm Hg [57, 261], the mucosal blood vessels become engorged, there are serous and/or hemorrhagic exudations into the ME cavity and, occasionally, the RW membrane may be ruptured [cf. chapter 7] [62, 124, 240, 272, 279]; furthermore, the TM is forced extremely far inward and may eventually be ruptured. *McGibbon* [279] found TM ruptures produced in this manner in 7 out of 100 cases of barotrauma caused during airplane flights; *King* [240] observed them in 38 out of a total of 897 cases. During diving, higher differential pressures are encountered. Among professional divers, because of their training, TM perforations are rare. Among amateur scuba divers, they may occur more frequently, but reliable statistics are not available.

King [241] and also *Love and Caruso* [272] described a delayed reaction that used to occur quite frequently in personnel who were breathing compressed air from a mask while flying nonpressurized aircraft. Under these conditions, the oxygen is quickly absorbed and, later on, quickly released. The nitrogen, however, is absorbed more slowly and released only after some delay. (Hence, this was only a problem of prolonged flights.) People thus exposed woke up in the middle of the night and had to clear their ears. However, since flying personnel as a rule have well-trained Eustachian tubes, no serious aftereffects have been reported [435].

A sudden increase of air pressure in the EEC may be produced by the pressure pulse of an explosion or a blow to the head closing off the canal entrance. The latter accident may lead to a blast injury in the following manner [75]: When the ear is hit by the palm of a hand or a ball, or when someone falls flat on the water surface, the pinna is flattened and its rims are sealed. The enclosed air (approximately 4.8 ml) is forced into the EEC that has only a volume of about 1.1 ml. By compressing a total volume of 5.9 ml into a space of 1.1 ml the pressure is increased by a factor of 5.4. That is to say, in reference to the normal atmospheric pressure, there is an increment of 4.4 atm. This increment exceeds by far the maximum the TM is able to withstand: 2,280 mm Hg, i.e. approximately 3 atm [473]. Consequently, the TM is ruptured. The extent of the lesion does not depend so much on the magnitude of the blow itself, but rather on the effectiveness of the object hitting the ear in sealing the pinna and thus in compressing the enclosed air.

Explosions produce TM ruptures mainly during wars. *Gruber* [155] was the first to describe such a lesion that he had seen after the battle of Sadowa (1866). Curiously, only a few such reports exist from the times of either world war [e.g. 225, 433]. This might have been related to the fact that, in these pretympanoplastic times, there was rarely any occasion for therapeutic intervention. *Korkis* [255] presented a relatively large collection of 167 cases. Later reports dealt mainly with incidental injuries caused by firework devices or incurred in industrial accidents. There are some contemporary reports stemming from recent military actions, e.g. in Northern Ireland [232, 336], in Egypt [393], in Israel [478], and in Vietnam [423].

Dietzel [75] was of the opinion that the TM may be damaged either by the initial, rapidly rising, positive pressure pulse or by the subsequent phase of negative pressure. *Kerr* [232], *Pahor* [336], and *Sudderth* [423], on the other hand, held mainly the initial pressure pulse responsible, the more so the longer its duration — up to a reported maximum of 1.5 msec — and the higher the peak pressure; the latter becomes especially high in enclosed spaces.

Kerr [232] observed, after an explosion taking place in a fully occupied restaurant, that, in contrast to the adults present, the children did not suffer any TM ruptures. This finding appears to confirm *Zalewski*'s [473] earlier experimental results, i.e. that the TM becomes more vulnerable with age.

It has been claimed that the ear that faces an explosion is most likely the one being damaged, whereas one that is covered by a turban or an earphone, is better protected [402].

Dietzel [75] found most posttraumatic perforations in the anteroinferior quadrant of the TM, as did *Passow* [339] before him. *Dietzel* [75] saw the explanation for this in the fact that the pressure pulse would act normal on this region of the TM — as does indeed a light beam going down the EEC. (This is not a very likely explanation as we shall see presently.)

Explosive devices of small yield (bazookas, for example) rupture the TM only when detonating close to the ear [255]. (This should also apply to the noise makers mentioned above [75].) Devices of larger yield, such as artillery shells, bombs, mines, on the other hand, produce damage even when distances are larger, i.e. up to 30 m. They are therefore responsible for most of the injuries observed [225, 255]. Furthermore, *Korkis* [255] did not find evidence indicating that the direction an explosive pulse came from determined which ear would be injured. Although the ipsilateral ear was more frequently involved, about one quarter of all injuries occurred bilaterally. *El Seifi* [393] found bilateral injuries in one third of his 108 cases. (Even in the open, the directional effect might be frequently obscured by reflections from various obstacles.)

The fact whether the mouth was open or closed at the time of an explosion does not matter either [255]. This finding excludes a potential role of the Eustachian tube. TM ruptures caused by explosions are preferentially located in the anteroinferior quadrant, never in Shrapnell's membrane [255].

Short-lasting positive pressure pulses, shorter than 1.5 msec, are thought to be mainly responsible for *inner*-ear lesions, while the TM would most likely be damaged by pulses lasting longer than 3–4 msec.

(These observations may be accounted for in terms of TM impedance. In a long-duration pulse, most of the energy is concentrated in the low-frequency region. While the reactive part of the TM impedance increases with inverse frequency — hence the TM displacements become large — little of that energy is transferred into the inner ear, since the resistive part, the only one capable of doing any work, is relatively small [500]. With short-duration pulses, the situation is reversed: the reactive part is small and the resistive one relatively larger. Hence, most of the incident energy is transferred into the inner ear and TM displacements do not become excessive.)

3.1.4. Lesions Caused by Blunt Head Trauma

Tears of the TM and of the fibrous annulus are frequently found as part of a longitudinal TB fracture spreading into the EEC [56, 105]. However, there are only a few cases on record in which a blunt head trauma led to a *central* perforation [352].

Armstrong [13] saw 57 TM ruptures. 10 of them were caused by blunt head injuries; no other details were given. *Escher* [102, 104] observed 3 TM ruptures in his 23 cases of longitudinal TB fractures (in addition to the other signs and symptoms seen); he gave no further details either. *Hartmann* [176], *Corradi* [63], as well as *Passow* [339] already knew that central perforations may occur in conjunction with a blunt head trauma. *Passow* thought that transient deformations of the tympanic ring, although not fracturing the bone, might rupture the TM, aided by the concomitant air pressure pulse.

3.2. Signs and Symptoms and Their Diagnostic Significance

Signs and symptoms of ME barotrauma not complicated by TM ruptures are easily accounted for on the basis of the etiology just described. A negative pressure existing in the ME causes shooting pains. The subsequent exudate produces a sensation of fullness in the ear, accompanied by some hearing loss [62, 70, 240, 272, 279]. Occasionally, there are complaints about tinnitus and/or dizziness [279]. Otoscopically, the TM appears whitish or livid. It is retracted and there is vascular injection. Pure-tone audiometry reveals a purely conductive hearing loss, exactly like that found with exudates of infectious origin. These signs and symptoms gradually subside as the serous-hemorrhagic exudate disappears. Its drainage may be accelerated by proper management of nasopharyngeal infections, if present; by decongestion of the tubal mucosa with the aid of topically applied antihistaminic and vasoconstricting agents; or by myringotomy [240, 272, 279].

Barotrauma, blast injuries and direct mechanical insults produce essentially the same type of central perforation. For the sake of the present discussion, they may therefore be lumped together. At the very beginning, the patient may notice a 'popping' sound [209, 339]. Later on, there is hearing loss and tinnitus. Occasionally, pain may be experienced and there may be bleeding from the ear [255]. (Bleeding occurs only when either the lining of the EEC or the ME mucosa are lacerated [209].) Otoscopy reveals a slit-like or triangular perforation, its edges being encrusted with blood. The apices of triangular perforations may point toward the umbo [473] or toward the annulus [75]. Some authors saw both forms [170].

As was repeatedly mentioned, the perforation is usually located in the anteroinferior quadrant when caused either by a barotrauma or a blast injury. Shrapnell's membrane is hardly ever involved [232, 255, 423, 473]. Multiple perforations are rarely seen [255, 273]. 4 separate perforations in 1 TM caused by one and the same explosion were described, but only once [209].

The rims of traumatic perforations tend to roll up or fold under on the ME side [219, 297]. After some time, they might adhere to the promontory or the incudostapedial joint [75].

Blast and/or mechanical injuries frequently carry foreign material into the ME: cerumen, pieces of epithelium, water or other matters. These materials usually produce inflammatory reactions [75, 423, 473, 480]. Hence, traumatic TM ruptures are often followed by acute otitis media [255, 402]. In the long run, the rolled-up edges may form a thickened ring of scar tissue, rendering the perforation round or kidney-shaped, essentially like that seen in a chronic suppurative otitis media [75, 99]. If deeply recessed into the ME, the rim of the perforation may attach itself permanently to the medial wall [75].

Strong and persistent dizzy spells following ME trauma are often signs of labyrinthine fistulae (cf. chapter 8). Perforations located in the posterosuperior quadrant should alert one to the possibility of an ossicular chain injury [13]. Piercing of the tympanic roof and subsequent cerebrospinal fluid (CSF) discharge are said to occur in conjunction with mechanical injuries of the TM, but are apparently rare [209, 382, 453].

As already stated, tuning-fork tests or pure-tone audiometry reveal purely conductive hearing losses. Covering the perforation should immediately improve hearing. If this does not occur, an ossicular-chain discontinuity should be suspected [221]. (For a detailed discussion cf. chapter 4.) Injuries caused by explosions [233, 366, 402, 423, 474] and by blunt head traumata [99, 118] often produce cochlear lesions, in addition to those of the ME.

Lesions caused by thermal injuries are also most frequently found in the anteroinferior quadrant [186, 371, 446]. As was already mentioned, the local heat effect rarely destroys all three TM layers at once, i.e. there is hardly ever a primary perforation. Initially, there may only be a third-degree burn. After a few days, the lacerated tissues are sloughed off, giving way to a perforation [371, 446]. The leading symptom is pain. The hearing loss may initially be slight. During the early stages, otoscopy reveals a TM that is deeply red and edematous. There may or may not be a perforation, but a foreign body may be lodged in the tissues. During the later stages, a strong watery discharge is quite characteristic. *Mosher* [313] assumed that this fluid discharge might often flush out the foreign body. Ultimately, a central perforation remains, round or kidney-shaped and framed by a ring of scar tissue. Ossicular lesions caused by pieces of hot metal have not been reported, although their incidence is quite conceivable. The occurrence of thermal lesions of the FN and of the cochlea were already mentioned in chapter 3.1.2.

Marginal perforations of the TM are produced by tears in the fibrous annulus in connection with longitudinal fractures of the TB. The main sign is a sanguinous discharge from the ear. Nevertheless, the other signs of longitudinal fractures, such as FN paralysis, CSF leakage, as well as the neurological signs and symptoms related to the underlying skull-brain trauma, are very much in the foreground and thus in the focus of interest (cf. chapter 6). Hence the tearing of the TM is initially of secondary importance.

Otitis media may follow, caused by the migration of bacteria into the damaged region [102, 285].

The understanding of the mechanisms underlying TM injuries has led, quite logically, to a postulate that was voiced by a number of authors in an almost identical manner [13, 75, 99, 151, 171, 287, 314]. All of them concluded that the proper diagnosis and management of such cases demand an exact otoscopic examination, including tuning-fork tests, pure-tone audiometry, trial covering of the perforation and a search for vestibular signs and symptoms.

3.3. Therapy

There are no firm guidelines for the management of marginal TM perforations caused by longitudinal TB fractures. It will be determined by the type and extent of the original injuries and their complications (cf. chapters 5, 6).

The presentation that follows deals therefore exclusively with the therapeutic measures recommended for *central* perforations of traumatic origin and with the results achieved.

3.3.1. Spontaneous Healing

Normal TM possess a strong potential for regeneration and self-repair. Animal experiments (cats [281, 356]; guinea pigs [355]) showed that even extensive defects produced experimentally healed spontaneously in most cases. As a rule, the repair started out from the squamous epithelium in the region of the annulus and in that of the umbo. When injured, this epithelium becomes very active, showing an increased number of mitoses and a tendency to proliferate in the general direction of the opposite wound margin. It literally pulls the granulation tissue of the middle layer along.

TM self-repair in the animals used in the above experiments is generally considered to be superior to that seen in humans [435]. However, clinical observations indicate that the human TM heals also quite well [339, 367]. This inherent potential, together with the fact that appropriate therapeutic measures were not available in the premicrosurgical era, originally fostered an attitude referred to as a 'watchful neglect' [56]. The ear was simply covered with sterile bandages and periodically inspected. Some authors recommended cleansing of the ear canal under aseptic conditions and pro-phylactic, systematic administration of antibiotics [283]. Rinsing out an in-jured ear was considered contraindicated [176, 339]. If there was otorrhea, the infection was treated by topical measures. Such superinfections were seen almost invariably after mechanical perforations, less frequently after simple ruptures [209].

Armstrong [13] considered the topical application of corticosteroids con-traindicated, since they might retard the spontaneous healing process. The application of eardrops of any kind when there are TM perforations can no longer be condoned. It was recently shown that many pharmaceutics not considered ototoxic, when applied directly into the ME, may diffuse through the RW membrane and thus damage the cochlea [34, 44, 48].

The spontaneous healing of TM perforations was aided by cauterization of its rims with the aid of trichloracidic acid [328, 331], cantharidin (*Baron* in discussion of [315], *Heermann*, cited after [170]) or silver nitrate [170] to stimulate the proliferation of granulation tissue. This was the only therapeu-tic measure employed.

Published papers differ widely with respect to the predicted rate of spontaneous closure of traumatic perforations and the time period required. *Wehmer* [458] went so far as to state that traumatic TM perforations should always heal, provided superinfections would not intervene. He considered failure of healing counterevidence against a traumatic origin. *Passow* [339] and *Imhofer* [209], on the other hand, saw persisting perforations, even when of proven traumatic origin. *Passow* [339] stated that, in a series of 25 trau-matic perforations he had seen (1 double perforation among them), 2 were still open after 5 years. According to *Imhofer*'s [209] accumulated statistics, the time required for spontaneous closure varied between 1 week (a case of *Passow*'s [339]) and 3–6 weeks. *McReynolds* et al. [283], out of a total of 77 traumatic perforations, all caused by explosions, found that 25 had healed spontaneously within the first 10 days. After 30 more days, 11 were still open. *Korkis* [255] was able to reexamine 70 ears out of a series of 167 with traumatically ruptured TM. After 69 days, all of them had healed. When no superinfections had intervened, healing, on the average, occurred faster (me-dian value: 29 days) than when there had been infections (median value: 38 days). *Herrmann* [191] saw 66 traumatic TM perforations; 28 of them still persisted after half a year. In his experience, the chances for spontaneous healing were the poorer, the larger the perforation. *El Seifi* [393] gave similar figures: in a group of 120 traumatic TM ruptures, only 49 had healed spontaneously within a period of 3 months. *Kerr* [233], on the other hand, found 55 that had healed spontaneously out of a total group of 66; all of them had been caused by one and the same explosion, i.e. by a bomb thrown into a restaurant (cf. above). *Singh and Ahluwalia* [402] treated 52 traumatically ruptured TM by conservative measures for a period of 4 weeks. During this period, 39 had healed, out of a group of 43, in whom the perforation had occupied less than one third of the TM area. Among the remaining 9, in whom the perforation had been larger, only 2 had healed. Table I presents a summary on these and other, additional observations; however, details on the origin of these lesions, their size, the duration of extended observations and the percentage of those reexamined are not included.

As table I shows, the median percentage of spontaneous healing was 73.7%, with extremes being as low as 41% and as high as 100%. The reports listed confirm the previous statement, i.e. that the tendency of the human TM to heal spontaneously is rather good and also that the chances of healing decrease with the size of the perforations as well as with the duration of their existence.

Ever since their first description by *Bezold* [30], it was recognized that *thermal* lesions of the TM do not heal well on their own. *Bezold* [30] saw 2 cases in which the TM perforations had been produced by scalding. He found their sizes to decrease during the early stages (in 1 of them, there was even a transient closure), but later on to increase once more. *Friedmann* (in

Table I. Spontaneous repair of the tympanic membrane (literature survey)

Author	Total number of cases	Healed	
		absolute figures	percentages
El Seifi [393]	120	49	41
Herrmann [191]	60	32	53
Kerr [233]	66	55	83
Korkis [255]	70	70	100
McReynolds et al. [283]	77	66	86
Mounier-Kuhn [315]	5	3	60
Pahor [336]	27	22	81
Passow [339]	25	23	92
Singh and Ahluwalia [402]	52	41	79
Ziv et al. [478]	60	53	88
Total	562	414	73.7

a discussion to [17]) described a spontaneous closure that occurred in a TM burned by molten iron. *Heermann* [186] found 4 TM that had healed spontaneously among the 15 cases he had collected. *Vick* [446] saw 2 out of a total of 34, *Mosher* [313] 9 out of 13. *Schein* [371], although not providing any details on his 44 cases, made the general statement, i.e. that the chances for spontaneous healing were poor if the size of the perforation exceeded one eighth of one TM quadrant. *Möbius* [304] reported spontaneous healing in 12 cases; in all of them the TM had allegedly been perforated during welding accidents; however, the cause had not been documented immediately after the accidents.

Individual reports on thermal TM lesions differ so widely from one another that reliable percentages cannot be given as to how many of them had spontaneously healed or not healed.

Summarizing at this point, we may quote *Escher* [99]: 'In contrast to perforations caused by blast injuries, chances for the spontaneous healing (of TM burns) are rather poor, on account of the scarring of their rims.'

3.3.2. Approximation of Wound Margins

The studies of *Lange* [262] demonstrated that the edges of a TM rupture usually fold under on the tympanic side, as was already mentioned. Thus, the free rims point away from one another, making spontaneous repair difficult. With the introduction of tympanoplastic procedures, otosurgeons began to inspect ruptured TM under the operating microscope, to remove debris and to unroll the folded-in sections. However, it turned out that after having been unrolled, the edges usually folded in once more. A solution to this problem had to be found. Methods suitable for aiding the epithelium to grow toward the opposite rim of a perforation, i.e. by putting some tissue on top of the TM, were known since the turn of the century. They were reintroduced in the 1950s [67, 328]. A suitable technique for fixing the TM edges was developed by *Hahlbrock* [170]. In 9 cases, in which the TM had been widely torn by explosions, he approximated the edges as best he could on top of some jelly enriched with penicillin. From all aspects, structural as well as functional, 7 of the 9 perforations he so treated healed well within periods of about 4 months. *Juers* [219], at about the same time, described an office procedure for the closing of central perforations of nontraumatic origin: he cauterized their rims and covered the defect by tissue paper. A short time later, he adapted this procedure to the case of perforations of traumatic origin [220].

These methods, i.e. (a) cleaning the middle ear under microscopic control, (b) unrolling the edges of the perforation, (c) approximating them over a jelly deposit, and (d) supporting the membrane by a cover on the canal side, were adopted by many other otosurgeons. However, different authors recommended different materials for the use as an outside support: *Hahl-brock* [170] employed his jelly also for this purpose or used nothing but the jelly deposit on the inside. This method was employed by *Herrmann* [191] as well as by *Goodhill* [140]. (The latter author recommended it also for stimu-lating TM repair after any other form of tympanoplasty.) *Juers* [221] used pieces of tissue paper slightly larger than the defect to be covered. *Langen-beck* [263] employed a mesh of cotton soaked in some ointment. *Dietzel* [75] used a silver-foil cover. *Dieroff* [74] applied sterilized egg membranes, *Escher* [98] silicone foils. Some authors preferred transparent materials, such as polyethylene foils (*Friedmann* in discussion to [191]), Scotch tape [194] or gelfilm [420, 478]. The question whether a fresh slice of garlic acts bacte-riostatically and thus promotes healing [207], or whether this is just another version of an old myth, i.e. that garlic put in the ear is good against earache [239], shall remain open.

The technical modifications described are most likely of secondary im-portance. What really matters is: the careful approximation of the edges of the perforation carried out under microscopic control and in local anesthesia (*Hahlbrock* [171] was the only one recommending general anesthesia); a suit-able fixation of the edges in their proper position, and timely administration of antibiotics to prevent infection. Table II summarizes the results obtained by following this regimen.

The results given in table II vary to a lesser extent than those achieved by waiting for spontaneous healing. Moreover, the median percentage value of success, 96%, is clearly higher than that of spontaneous closures, 73.3%. This comparison demonstrates the efficacy of active intervention.

A paper by *Ziv* et al. [478] is of special interest in this connection. These authors were able to examine two rather homogeneous groups of patients injured in two separate accidents: (a) from a destroyer sunk at sea, and (b) from a truck that, being loaded with explosives, had blown up. There were 60 TM ruptures in the first group. All of them were treated by conservative measures. 7 perforations remained open (11.6%). In the second group, there were 22 TM ruptures. Active intervention with approximation of the edges of the perforation led to the closure of all but 1 of them (4.5%).

Audiometric results after surgical intervention are quite good, according to the various authors cited. Several of them, however, suggested that one

Table II. Tympanic membrane repair after wound approximation (literature survey)

Author	Number of cases	Healed		Method employed
		absolute figures	percentages	
Hahlbrock [171]	9	7	78	jelly plug
Weilepp and Rentzsch [459]	102	99	97	cotton-ointment
Dietzel [75]	57	52	91	cotton-oinment and silver foil
Juers [221]	90	89	99	tissue paper
El Seifi [393]	28	25	89	jelly plug
Herrmann [191]	11	11	100	jelly plug
Armstrong [13]	57	57	100	jelly plug
Oppenheimer et al. [333]	12	12	100	jelly plug
Ziv et al. [478]	22	21	95	gelfilm
Mostafa [314]	20	19	95	jelly plug
Strebel [420]	32	31	97	gelfilm
Total	440	423	96	

should wait for about 3 weeks after surgery before retesting a patient's hearing. It would take that much time until the jelly deposit in the ME had sufficiently liquefied and drained via the Eustachian tube. *Weilepp and Rentzsch* [459] presented their audiometric findings in quite some detail. They were able to follow-up on 102 patients. 5–6 weeks after the termination of treatment, 76.9% of them showed audiometric improvements, 12.9% further deterioration and 10.2% no changes. On reexamination, 2.5–5 years later, these values had changed to 84.7, 10.2 and 5.1%, respectively.

TM burns are in a class by themselves. The edges of the perforation cannot be approximated, since the tissue necrosis left a true defect. One may of course cover it in an effort to guide the proliferating tissues, yet the chances for spontaneous healing are still poor, as was already mentioned. *Vick* [446] successfully closed 6 out of 34 such defects by covering them with cotton soaked in some ointment.

3.3.3. Tympanoplasty

Opinions differ widely as to the chances of successfully closing posttraumatic TM perforations with the aid of tympanoplastic procedures. As already mentioned, a perforation that does not heal on its own acquires, in the long run, the shape of a central perforation, essentially like that seen in chronic otitis media. That is to say, its edges that initially were multifaceted and might have included some irregular small flaps are rounded off, forming a tight ring of scar tissue. Even at this stage, some authors still prefer conservative measures, i.e. to cauterize or deepithelialize the edges and to cover the perforation from the outside [328]. More recently, however, otologists tend toward surgical closure of persistent perforations. *Hahlbrock* [171] advocated tympanoplasty when a perforation had persisted for more than 3 months. *Singh and Ahluwalia* [402] performed surgery already after 3–4 weeks; *Sudderth* [423] advocated surgery when coverage by tissue paper failed to promote healing, although he gave no time limits. *Khan* [237] recommended early intervention in every case, *Silverstein* et al. [397] even within the first 48 h.

Armstrong [13] advocated an early exploratory tympanotomy if the location of the perforation — especially when in the posterosuperior quadrant — or other details suggest either damage to the ossicular chain or the presence of a foreign body. Following his own recommendations, he carried out a total of 57 tympanotomies and found positive results in 20 of them. (Some indications with regard to the presence of concomitant ossicular chain lesions may be obtained from a trial covering of the perforation [220], as was already mentioned.) *Boenninghaus* [37], on the other hand, does not consider tympanoplasty unless surgical intervention is required on account of grave injuries to the base of the temporal bone.

Only a few statistics are available on the outcome of surgical closure of posttraumatic TM perforations. They are given in table III.

It was not surprising that results were less successful after tympanoplasty than after simple wound approximation. For one thing, the total number of cases reported is relatively small, i.e. only 177, thus making the evidence statistically uncertain. Secondly, the above comparison gives a one-sided story: tympanoplasty was performed only when there were large defects present and/or when spontaneous healing had failed to take place. Thirdly, some of the poor results reported ought to be charged to the surgical techniques employed. The 5 recurring perforations reported by *Silverstein* et al. [397] may serve as an example: In 1 of them, only gelfoam was put in on the tympanic side; in another, amnion was used, but it was put on the outside, and, in the 3 remaining cases, fascia was employed in the same manner. In all cases that had healed well, fat tissue or fascia had been put on the *tympanic* side. *Sudderth* [423], when placing fascia on the tympanic side, had poor results in only 2 out of 45 cases (4.5%) so treated. When placing it on

Table III. Tympanic membrane ruptures repaired by tympanoplasty (literature survey)

Author	Number of cases	Healed		Method employed
		absolute figures	percentages	
Khan [237]	28	28	100	homologous fascia medially and canal skin externally
Ruggles and Votypka [336]	11	7	64	gelfoam (6 times) fascia (5 times)
Silverstein et al. [397]	20	15	75	fat tissue or fascia
Singh and Ahluwalia [402]	11	9	82	vein
Sudderth [423]	107	92	86	fascia, partly medially, partly externally
Total	177	151	85.3	

the canal side, however, he obtained poor results in 13 out of 45 cases that included 4 cholesteatomata. One must therefore agree with *Khan*'s [237] statement, i.e. that the chances for success are best when one places some material on the tympanic side of the TM, preferably in conjunction with some outer cover on the canal side.

With respect to the tympanoplastic procedures required, TM burns once more present a special problem. Large defects with scarred rims do require surgical repair. A number of authors demand that the ear be completely dry before surgery, i.e. that active infections should no longer exist, that necrotic tissue, if still present, should be clearly demarkated and finally, that one should not operate too soon after the original injury. *Frenkiel and Alberti* [133] prefer to wait for several months. *Vick* [446] turns to surgery only after all conservative measures have been exhausted. *Grimaud* et al. [151] demand that the ear in question should not have shown any secretion for at least 6 months. Otherwise, all authors, who described their procedures in detail, adhere to general tympanoplastic principles. The materials preferred include autologous fascia [288, 411], Thiersch grafts [288], perichondrium [151] or homologous TM [151].

The results achieved by the various authors listed are compiled in table IV. Table IV includes 3 cases of scalding of the TM — one each of *Kuruma* et al. [258], *Martin* et al. [288], and *Sprem* [411]. All of them had healed

Table IV. Thermal injuries, repaired by tympanoplasty (literature survey)

Author	Number of cases	Healed		Method employed
		absolute figures	percentages	
Frenkiel and Alberti [133]	8	3	38	—
Grimaud et al. [151]	8	5	63	perichondrium, homologous tympanic membrane (twice)
Kuruma et al. [258]	1	1	100	—
Martin et al. [288]	8	5	63	fascia or Thiersch graft
Sprem [411]	1	1	100	fascia
Vick [446]	28	22	79	—
Total	54	37	68.5	

well. All other injuries stemmed from industrial accidents and were mostly caused by welding sparks. The total rate of success, 68.5%, was clearly less than that obtained, also by tympanoplastic procedures, but in patients with simple TM ruptures, i.e. 85.3%.

3.4. Present Study: Clinical Findings and Postmortem Results

A total of 500 patients with TM injuries were studied. Since 31 of them had *bilateral* lesions, the number of ears involved was 531. All perforations were located in pars tensa, none of them in pars flaccida. Single perforations were present in 524 ears. There were 5 double perforations (4 of them caused by slaps on the ear, 1 by an explosion) and 2 triple perforations (in 1 case, they were produced by instrumental cleaning of the EEC and were located anteroposteriorly, posteroinferiorly, and the third between these 2; in the other, the cause was not specified). In the following, the multiple perforations will be listed as if they were single. Their locations will be given as that of the largest one.

3.4.1. Causes
The causes of all 531 perforations are listed in table V, the total being set at 100%.

Table V. Causes of 531 tympanic membrane ruptures

	Number of cases	Percentages	
Direct traumata	448	84.5	
Explosions	110	21 ⎫	Blast traumata
Slaps on the ear	143	27 ⎬	[n = 303 (57.5%)]
Swimming accidents	50	9.5 ⎭	
Barotraumata	22	4	
Mechanical cleaning of ear canal	37	7 ⎫	Mechanical traumata
Foreign bodies	29	5.5 ⎬	[n = 83 (15.5%)]
Irrigations of ear canal	17	3 ⎭	
Thermal traumata	21	4	
Causes not given	19	3.5	
Skull injuries	83	15.5	
After falling or being hit	42	8	
Traffic accidents	37	7	
Gunshot injuries	3	0.5	
Causes not given	1	—	

This compilation indicates that the majority, i.e. 84.5% of the lesions, resulted from direct injuries to the TM. These were far more numerous than indirect injuries produced in the course of blunt head traumata. More than one half of the total, i.e. 57.5%, were caused by blast injuries, only 4% by barotraumata. Mechanical injuries and indirect injuries associated with blunt head traumata were equal in frequency of occurrence, each accounting for 15.5%. A detailed analysis of 78 blast-induced TM ruptures with known causes is presented in table VI.

The toy balloons listed were either filled with ordinary household gas or with acetylene. Most of them had exploded in batches, although sequentially, while being transported. Table VI indicates that accidents caused by toys (38.5%) outnumbered those occurring in industry (16.5%). Injuries produced by weapons had been sustained during either of the two world wars or they were incurred by foreign nationals who were involved in military actions in their home countries. It goes without saying that the incidence of such injuries would have been much higher at times of war.

Blows to the ear were either caused by a hand or by some mechanical instrument, such as a ball. The mechanism underlying these injuries was the air-volume compression in the EEC already described [75]. Some patients, of course, denied having been slapped, inventing some other cause instead.

Table VI. Detailed analysis of 78 injuries caused by explosions

	Number of cases		
Noise makers	12	Toy	n = 30 (38.5%)
Toy balloons	18		
Gas explosions	7	Professional accidents	n = 13 (16.5%)
Blasting	6		
Blank ammunition	2		
Hand guns	2		
Hand grenades	3		
Artillery shells	9	War-related injuries	n = 35 (45%)
Bombs	4		
Mines	13		
Rockets	2		

TM ruptures caused by swimming accidents, i.e. when somebody was jumping into the water or was hit under water, were considered as separate entities, although some of these ruptures might have been produced by *Dietzel*'s [75] air-compression mechanism. However, when the EEC was filled with water both cause and effect could have been different.

The perforations produced by water pressure do not look like traumatic ruptures at all. They are roundish and the rims are usually not encrusted by blood. Cadaver experiments revealed that, in contrast to air entrapped in the EEC, the incompressible water gradually forces its way in between the TM fibers, simply pressing them aside. The water does not expand explosively the moment the TM yields [494].

Included under the heading of barotrauma were 21 typical TM ruptures found in divers. One other rupture was produced during the nose dive of an airplane, a finding that confirmed the theoretical considerations of chapter 3.1.3.

Both instrumental cleaning attempts and foreign bodies entering the EEC led to direct mechanical injuries. For the following reasons, however, one must consider these two modes of injury separately: When intending to clean an EEC one introduces an instrument deliberately, and it is usually fairly clean. After an injury has occurred, the instrument is invariably, and usually quickly, withdrawn. A foreign body, on the other hand, gets into the EEC, either accidentally or, in children, during play. More often than not, it is dirty and remains in the EEC for an extended period of time, often even behind a perforated TM. Therefore, posttraumatic infections, or at least

Table VII. Instruments used for the cleaning of ear canals and removal of foreign bodies

	Cases
Cleaning of the ear canal (n = 32)	
Q-Tip	29
Match	2
Wooden stick	1
Foreign bodies with tympanic	
membrane perforations (n = 22)	
Small twig	5
Wooden stick	4
Piece of straw	2
Pussy willow	2
Pieces of metal	2
Copper wire	1
Knitting needle	1
Sharp handle of comb	1
Metal nail	1
Pipette (for ear drops)	1
Pebble	1
Wheat kernel	1
Foreign bodies located in middle ear (n = 4)	
Matches	2
Pencil lead	1
Piece of straw	1

delays in healing, are more likely to occur with foreign bodies than after instrumental cleaning attempts. Table VII lists the devices and objects, as far as they could be determined, that had produced TM ruptures by mechanical means.

In only 1 of the cases listed was the TM perforation suspected of having been caused by a misguided attempt to extract a foreign body. In all others, they had been produced directly by the foreign body itself.

3.4.2. Distribution by Age, Sex and Sidedness

TM injuries were seen in a total of 500 persons, 345 men and 155 women. Table VIII shows the age distribution of these persons at the time the injuries were sustained. The table is subdivided into 13 categories, i.e. 12 different causes plus the total. (1 additional case of head trauma is not listed, since no detailed information could be obtained.)

Table VIII. Tympanic membrane injuries of various causes in 500 cases

Cause	Number of cases	Age, years							
		0–10 (%)	11–20 (%)	21–30 (%)	31–40 (%)	41–50 (%)	51–60 (%)	61–70 (%)	71–80 (%)
Total	500	46 (9)	120 (24)	163 (32.5)	98 (20)	44 (9)	13 (2.5)	13 (2.5)	3 (0.5)
1 Explosion	85	—	23 (27)	41 (48)	13 (15)	4 (5)	1 (1)	2 (2)	1 (1)
2 Slap on the ear	142	1 (1)	51 (36)	43 (30)	29 (20)	15 (10.5)	2 (1.5)	1 (1)	—
3 Swimming accident	49	2 (4)	14 (28.5)	23 (47)	5 (10.5)	4 (8)	1 (2)	—	—
4 Barotrauma	19	—	2 (10.5)	9 (47)	7 (37)	1 (5.5)	—	—	—
5 Instrumental cleaning of ear canal	37	21 (56.5)	4 (11)	6 (16)	2 (5.5)	2 (5.5)	2 (5.5)	—	—
6 Foreign body	29	12 (41)	6 (21)	3 (10.5)	5 (17)	2 (7)	—	1 (3.5)	—
7 Irrigation of ear canal	17	—	—	3 (17.5)	5 (30)	3 (17.5)	3 (17.5)	3 (17.5)	—
8 Thermal injury	21	—	—	3 (14)	13 (62)	4 (19)	1 (5)	—	—
9 After falling or being hit	41	3 (7)	4 (10)	10 (24)	12 (29)	6 (15)	1 (2.5)	4 (10)	4 (2.5)
10 Traffic accident	37	4 (11)	11 (30)	11 (30)	5 (14)	1 (2.5)	2 (5)	2 (5)	1 (2.5)
11 Gunshot injury	3	—	—	3	—	—	—	—	—
12 No details given	19	3 (16)	5 (26)	7 (37)	2 (10.5)	2 (10.5)	—	—	—

As indicated, about three quarters of all injuries occurred between the 11th and 40th years of life. The exceptions were: (a) the injuries produced by cleaning of the EEC and by foreign bodies (they were prevalent in children below the age of 10), (b) those caused by falling, by being beaten and in traffic accidents (they were found mainly in children and in older people), and (c) thermal injuries (they occurred mainly in industry and were most frequent between the ages of 21 and 50).

The distribution by sex and by sideness is given in table IX. Table IX shows that women suffered TM injuries less frequently than men. This was correct both for the total group as well as for the separate categories. The difference was especially large with respect to accidents (explosions, barotraumata, thermal injuries, swimming pool accidents, traffic accidents). That it was likewise so for blows to the ear was contrary to the finding of other authors [e.g. 480]. Women, when falling, sustained TM injuries nearly as frequently as men because of the high incidence of domestic accidents. Instrumental cleaning and irrigation of the EEC caused even more TM injuries in women than in men.

That the *left* TM was more frequently injured by slaps on the ear is explained by the fact that most people when slapping others use their right hand. Since welders lean their heads slightly toward the right while working, their left TM were also more frequently injured than their right ones, a finding that had been made by others before [313, 371, 446]. No plausible explanation can be offered for the difference in sideness found in injuries produced when the EEC was being washed out. In all other categories the frequency of occurrence was about the same for the 2 ears.

Bilateral TM lacerations, as might be expected, were found frequently after explosions (29%) and also after barotrauma (16%). In both cases, the 2 ears are affected in essentially the same manner. After blunt skull trauma, bilateral injuries were rare, supporting an earlier assumption [84], i.e. that maximal damage is restricted to the region directly exposed to the trauma.

The following remarks apply to both tables VIII and IX: Although it represents a direct, mechanical injury, irrigation of the EEC with water is listed as a separate category. This was done in an effort to point out that this method, usually considered innocuous, may lead to TM injuries when performed in a careless manner. Moreover, if the TM is ruptured, water must certainly enter the ME, inviting infections that might delay healing. It is highly unlikely that these ruptures occurred only in ears, in which monomeric membranes had been present. In fact, it was only in 1 patient that the TM was noted to show scars from past infections.

The thermal trauma category included 1 case of scalding, but there was no information as to the size of the perforation produced. TM burns were seen in 20 cases; they had been caused by sparks originating from metal-

Table IX. Tympanic membrane injuries of various causes: distribution by sex and sidedness in 500 persons

Cause	Number of cases	Male	Female	M:F ratio	Right	Left	R:L ratio	Bilateral	%
Total	500	345	155	7:3	206	263	2:3	31	6
1 Explosion	85	80	5	9:1	34	26	3:2	25	29
2 Slap on the ear	142	86	56	6:4	44	97	3:7	1	0.7
3 Swimming accident	49	38	11	8:2	24	24	1:1	1	2
4 Barotrauma	19	15	4	8:2	8	8	1:1	3	16
5 Instrumental cleaning of the ear canal	37	17	20	5:5	19	18	1:1	—	—
6 Foreign body	29	19	10	7:4	16	13	6:5	—	—
7 Irrigation of ear canal	17	8	9	1:1	6	11	4:7	—	—
8 Thermal injury	21	21	—	10:0	8	13	4:6	—	—
9 After falling or being hit	41	23	18	6:4	19	21	1:1	1	2.5
10 Traffic accident	37	24	13	7:4	17	20	1:1	—	—
11 Gunshof injury	3	3	—	—	1	2	1:2	—	—
12 Ear injury, no details given	19	11	8	6:4	9	10	1:1	—	—
13 Skull trauma, (details not known)	1	—	1	—	1	—	—	—	—

grinding or welding operations or by pieces of flying cinder. In 1 more case, not listed here, the remnant of a burn was found on the malleus handle. Its cause was a welding accident, but it had apparently not led to a TM perforation. A concomitant lesion of the skin of the EEC was only seen in the patient with the scalding injury and in another with a welding-spark injury. In all others, hot particles had apparently passed through the EEC without touching its walls. In 2 patients injured during welding operations, X-ray pictures demonstrated a piece of metal lying in the ME. 1 of these patients refused surgery. In the other, it was eventually found lying between the promontory and the anterior stapedial crus, 10 full years after the original accident.

The blunt head traumata were divided into two subgroups: (a) those caused by falling or by being beaten, and (b) those incurred in traffic accidents. The latter category turned out to be rather small (7% of the total). Hence, the increase in the number of motor vehicles during the past decades had apparently not contributed to a higher incidence of TM lesions — at least not in the FRG.

All three gunshot injuries observed stemmed from the time of WW II. At that time, this type of injury must have been much more frequent, like that due to explosions.

19 patients could not be fitted into the classifications of tables VIII and IX because their past histories did not provide sufficient information. This introduced some uncertainty in these tables (and also into table X below). The size of this group was relatively large in comparison to that of the other categories. This shortcoming had to do with the fact that patients, in their critical conditions after head trauma, were difficult to examine.

2 of the patients with injuries caused by welding sparks presented in the clinic immediately after the accident. In both of them a foreign body of minute size was seen lodged in a reddened and thickened TM. It took 2 days until a perforation appeared at the site of the original lesion.

3.4.3. Location of Tympanic Membrane Perforations: Clinical Patients

All perforations were located in pars tensa, as was already mentioned. In the tables below, their exact sites are given in terms of the conventional division of the TM into quadrants. If the perforation went beyond the confines of one quadrant, it was considered to belong to that quadrant, in which its extent was largest. A perforation extending over more than one half of the TM area was classified as a subtotal defect.

The locations of all TM perforations are listed in table X. The two marginal perforations, mentioned in a footnote to categories 9 and 10, were real-

Table X. Location of 531 tympanic membrane perforations

Cause	Number of cases	Location					Details on location missing (%)
		ant.-sup. (%)	ant.-inf. (%)	post.-sup. (%)	post.-inf. (%)	subtotal (%)	
Total	531	42 (8)	236 (44)	49 (9)	85 (16)	46 (9)	69 (13)
1 Explosion	110	5 (4.5)	45 (41)	5 (4.5)	12 (11)	30 (27)	13 (12)
2 Slap on the ear	143	12 (8.5)	73 (51)	18 (12)	27 (19)	2 (1.5)	11 (8)
3 Swimming accident	50	7 (14)	25 (50)	2 (4)	10 (20)	2 (4)	4 (8)
4 Barotrauma	22	2 (9)	7 (32)	—	7 (32)	1 (4.5)	5 (22.5)
5 Instrumental cleaning of ear	37	1 (3)	14 (38)	9 (24)	10 (27)	—	3 (8)
6 Foreign body	29	1 (3)	13 (45)	4 (14)	4 (14)	3 (10)	4 (14)
7 Irrigation of ear canal	17	1 (6)	10 (59)	—	1 (6)	1 (6)	4 (23)
8 Thermal injury	21	2 (9.5)	13 (62)	1 (5)	—	2 (9.5)	3 (14)
9 After falling or being hit	42*	7 (16.5)	16 (38)	5 (12)	3 (7)	1 (2.5)	8 (19)
10 Traffic accident	37*	2 (5.5)	13 (35)	3 (8)	5 (13.5)	1 (2.5)	11 (30)
11 Gunshot injury	3	—	—	—	1 (33)	1 (33)	1 (33)
12 No details given	19	1 (5.5)	7 (37)	2 (10.5)	5 (26)	2 (10.5)	2 (10.5)
13 Skull trauma (details not known)	1	1	—	—	—	—	—

* Including 2 marginal perforations

ly extensions of fracture lines running along the posterior wall of the EEC. Such ruptures that are actually tears are typically associated with longitudinal TB fractures [105]; they are usually located in the posterosuperior quadrant of the TM. In the present total of 79 TM injuries caused by blunt head trauma (category 13) they were rather rare.

Central perforations were found in 42 cases but, except for the 2 cases just mentioned, there were no recognizable tears in the fibrous annulus. In 14 other cases, in which longitudinal fractures of the posterior canal wall could be demonstrated either by the presence of an osseous step, on X-ray pictures or during surgery, there were also central perforations, 4 times in the anterosuperior quadrant, 7 times in the anteroinferior, twice in the posterosuperior and once in the posteroinferior quadrants. However, no communication with the fracture lines could be demonstrated.

The location of the ruptures was relatively constant throughout the various categories of table X. The anteroinferior quadrant was most frequently involved, i.e. in 44% of all cases. If one leaves out the 19 patients for whom information was lacking, the percentage increases to even 51%. Next in order of the frequency of involvement was the posteroinferior quadrant, followed by the posterosuperior and, finally, the anterosuperior quadrant. The preference of thermal injuries for the anteroinferior quadrant is striking. Although the underlying mechanisms are certainly not identical, this was also the most frequent site of ruptures caused by blast trauma (explosions, slaps on the ear, barotrauma and swimming accidents: 46% of the total) and of those caused by direct mechanical injury (mechanical cleaning or irrigation of the EEC and foreign bodies: 45% of the total).

3.4.4. Location of Tympanic Membrane Perforations: Postmortem Specimens

Of the 89 TB made available for study, 1 was damaged during its removal, in 1 a chronic otitis media existed and in a third there was an old mastoidectomy cavity. In the remaining 86 TB, the condition of the TM could be evaluated. The results are presented in table XI.

In 18 of these TB, a longitudinal fracture was present. In 5 of the 18, the roof of the EEC was torn off by the fracture. The soft tissue lining of the EEC as well as Shrapnell's membrane were attached to the fragment. The TM was torn along the anterior and posterior mallar ligaments, but the pars tensa as such was intact. In 2 other cases, the fracture had split the EEC in its posterosuperior region. An osseous step had formed and the soft tissues over it were torn. Starting from the fracture line, a tear ran through the fibrous an-

Table XI. Tympanic membrane findings in 89 postmortem specimens

Evaluation of tympanic membrane possible in	Number of cases (n = 86)
Longitudinal fractures	18
Roof of external canal and Shrapnell's membrane torn off	5
Post.-sup. marginal perforation	2
Tympanic membrane intact	11
Central perforation —fibrous annulus intact	3
In ant.-inf. quadrant	2
In post.-sup. quadrant	1

nulus in a radial direction toward the umbo. In the remaining 10 cases of longitudinal fractures, the TM and the soft tissue lining of the EEC were intact.

Central perforations were found in 3 cases. All of them were fresh, i.e. caused by a recent trauma, as indicated by their sharp and partially rolled-up edges and by the presence of newly coagulated blood. 2 of the perforations were located in the anteroinferior quadrant. 1 had occurred in conjunction with a depressed fracture of the floor of the EEC, which had left the tympanic ring intact. The second was associated with a homolateral, frontobasal skull injury. The third perforation, located in the posterosuperior quadrant, accompanied a homolateral skull-base fracture in the posterior fossa.

3.4.5. Therapeutic Results: Influence of Causes and Specific Therapies

Minute slit-like perforations did not require any treatment, and there were several patients who refused treatment. One may safely assume that quite a number of patients with small perforations, but without superinfections, were taken care of by their private otologists on an outpatient basis so that they do not appear in the present survey. On the other hand, a fairly large number of patients were referred to the university hospitals because their perforations were of long standing, resisting any conservative therapy. It is for these reasons that the incidence of spontaneous closure given below is only representative of a secondary or even tertiary care hospital. For the general population, the rate should be much higher.

Active, local therapy, for the sake of simplicity, referred to as 'surgical measures', included the following:

(1) Fresh, noninfected perforations were covered by a piece of cigarette paper soaked in antibiotic ointment, provided the edges were not rolled in.

This mode of therapy was occasionally employed even with small perforations of some standing, after the rims had been cauterized by means of trichloracidic acid.

(2) Edges that were rolled up or small flaps that were folded in were straightened out in local anesthesia and approximated with the opposite side over a small piece of *gelita* laid down in the tympanic cavity. On the outside, the TM was covered by a silicone foil and a piece of gelfoam. This procedure was carried out in the operating room under sterile conditions and microscopic control; however, neither the EEC nor the ME were surgically explored.

(3) When there were extensive tissue defects or old perforations surrounded by scarred rims, or when injuries to other ME structures were suspected, the ME was explored either from the EEC or from a retroauricular approach. The continuity of the ossicular chain and the round window reflex were tested. Finally, a piece of fresh autologous fascia, or a homologous one preserved in *cialit,* according to the method of *Hildmann and Steinbach* [193], was positioned *under* the TM. Occasionally, the graft was fixed to the TM by pulling an edge of them through a small slit of the TM or a small piece of skin taken from the anterior part of the EEC was put onto the outside of the TM, followed by the usual silicone foil and pieces of gelfoam.

(4) If one or more ossicles were damaged, or if there were secondary changes in cases of long standing, the ossicular chain was reconstructed. The methods employed will be described in detail in chapter 4.4.2. In all these cases, the perforation was closed by a piece of fascia as described above under item (3).

The following measures may therefore be compared: (1) waiting for spontaneous closure; (2) covering the perforation from the outside and, if indicated, cauterization of its rims; (3) wound approximation; (4) tympanoplasty type I, and (5) (lumped together) tympanoplasty types II–IV.

A preliminary evaluation of results, subdivided into two groups: (1) spontaneous healing, and (2) all active measures taken together, is given in table XII.

The third column, labeled 'not healed', meant that there was no spontaneous healing. The fourth column, labeled 'late surgery', implied that active surgical intervention was undertaken when, and only when, there were no signs of spontaneous closure after a waiting period of at least 7 days; the fifth column, 'early surgery', that the surgeon intervened actively already during the first week, without waiting for spontaneous healing. Therefore no conclusions can be drawn from the percentages given in table XII with respect to the rate of spontaneous closures. A number of perforations subjected to early

Table XII. Tympanic membrane perforations: spontaneously healed, not healed, and surgical measures taken (early or late)

Cause	Total number of injuries	Spontaneously healed (%)	Not healed (%)	Late surgery (%)	Early surgery (%)
Total	531	62 (11.5)	88 (17)	183 (34.5)	198 (37)
1 Explosion	110	11 (10)	26 (24)	45 (41)	28 (25)
2 Slap on the ear	143	12 (8)	17 (12)	47 (33)	67 (47)
3 Swimming accident	50	5 (10)	9 (18)	16 (32)	20 (40)
4 Barotrauma	22	3 (14)	5 (23)	8 (36)	6 (27)
5 Instrumental cleaning of the ear canal	37	7 (19)	4 (11)	1 (2.5)	25 (67.5)
6 Foreign body	29	5 (17)	2 (7)	10 (34.5)	12 (41.5)
7 Irrigation of ear canal	17	1 (6)	6 (35)	7 (41)	3 (18)
8 Thermal injury	21	3 (14)	4 (19)	12 (57)	2 (10)
9 After falling or being hit	42	5 (12)	5 (12)	14 (33)	18 (43)
10 Traffic accident	37	9 (24)	4 (11)	14 (38)	10 (27)
11 Gunshot injury	3	0	1 (33)	2 (66)	0
12 No details given	19	1 (5)	5 (26)	6 (32)	7 (37)
13 Skull trauma (details not known)	1	0	0	1	0

surgery and even some of those undergoing late surgery might conceivably have healed spontaneously later on.

The significance of table XII lies in the *relative* rate of spontaneous closures with respect to the various causes listed. In the first four groups of pressure-induced trauma, the rates of spontaneous healing were approximately the same. Especially noted must be the fact that the rate was not poorer in the group of swimming accidents, although water might have entered the ME. However, when water was directly injected into the ME while the EEC was being irrigated in the presence of a TM perforation, the chances of spontaneous healing were definitely poor, i.e. only 6%.

The results found after instrumental cleaning attempts and after the intrusion of foreign bodies were in close agreement, indicating that the danger of contaminated material brought into the ME by a foreign body was not as severe as originally thought.

Somewhat unexpected, in view of the results published by others, was the high rate of spontaneous healing seen after welding accidents; with 14%, they were better than average. This finding may be related to the fact that early surgery was rarely performed on these lesions, i.e. in only 10% of them. Usually, a longer waiting period was kept. The figure of 14% given for this category may therefore be rather close to the general rate of spontaneous healing. However, this would not be true for those groups in which surgery was carried out routinely at an early stage. Similar considerations might help to explain the differences between categories 10 (12%) and 11 (24%). They might also be due to the choice of the time at which surgery was carried out. Early surgery was done in only 27% of the traffic accidents, presumably because other, more serious injuries had to be taken care of first; it was carried out in 43% of patients who had fallen or had been beaten.

The large number of TM ruptured by explosions, in which surgery was performed late, may be surprising. This was simply due to the fact that 45% of these ruptures had occurred during WW II, and that most of the patients did not present themselves earlier. This high rate of injuries of long standing shifted the relation between spontaneous healing and late surgery in favor of the latter category. Finally, the high rate of surgery performed early in the group of direct mechanical injuries, caused by cleaning attempts of the EEC, is accounted for by the fact that many of the ME involved had to be explored surgically to exclude lesions to the ossicular chain.

Some notion on the expected rate of spontaneous healing of TM perforations may be obtained when one determines for a number of subsequent time periods the ratio of healed perforations to those still persisting (regardless of whether these were later on operated or not). Table XIIIa presents the results together for all groups. (Subdivision by the various categories would have yielded numbers too small to be of any significance.) Nevertheless, in each individual category, the time period after injury was determined, during

Table XIIIa. Fate of tympanic membrane perforations over time

	Duration					
	0–1 weeks	1–3 weeks	4–6 weeks	7–13 weeks	4–6 months	> 6 months
A Healed spontaneously (n = 62)	3	19	14	12	4	10
B Not healed (n = 271)	46	30	18	24	16	137
C Spontaneous healings as percentages of A + B, % (Total: 19%)	6	39	44	33	20	7
Total number of perforations		531				
Healed spontaneously		62				
Not healed spontaneously		271				
Never healed		89				
Healed after late surgery		182				
Healed after early surgery		198				

which spontaneous healing occurred most frequently, and the rate prevailing during that period. Mean values and ranges of variation are presented in table XIIIb.

In the category of gunshot injuries the rate of spontaneous healing was zero, simply because all cases were of long standing. Table XIIIa indicates that some spontaneous closures occurred already during the first week after injury, a finding that confirms *Passow*'s [339] earlier notions. Nevertheless, the rate of spontaneous closure in table XIIIa did not become maximal until the fourth- to sixth-week period. The ratio of spontaneously healed ears (44%) might be fairly close to that occurring in a larger population, since a relatively large number of healed perforations as well as persisting ones happened to exist during that particular period. However, the point must be stressed again that the present survey is limited to patients seen at a university hospital; that is to say, cases without complications were probably encountered less frequently than they would have been in the population at large. It might be for the same reason that the ratio of healed perforations to those still persisting decreased noticeably after the sixth week, although even as late as 6 months after the injury some TM still healed spontaneously. As the time after injury progressed, new cases were added to the total group monitored by the department from an outside pool of old persisting perforations, but there were hardly any in which spontaneous healing could have been expected. The only conclusion that is really warranted on the basis of the present material is that the rate of spontaneous closure of ruptured TM is most likely higher than 44%, an order of magnitude that is also suggested by the findings of others ([191] 53%; [315] 60%; [393] 41%).

The percentage figures of spontaneous closure presented in table XIIIb are rendered somewhat uncertain in a statistical sense by the smallness of the absolute numbers. The significance of the table lies merely in pinpointing the time period, in which most spontaneous closures occurred. If in any given group the maximal value happens to coincide with the median, the distribution is symmetrical. If not, it is skewed. Inspection of table XIIIb indicates that the two values coincided in all categories; hence, that the distributions were symmetrical. For categories 2 and 3 (slap on the ear and swimming accidents) on the one hand and for categories 5 and 6 (direct

Table XIIIb. Fate of tympanic membrane perforations: time and ratio of spontaneous healing vs. overall spontaneous healing

Cause	Best spontaneous healing ratio, %	Time after injury	Medium time	Minimal to maximal time
1 Explosion	75	7 weeks to 6 months	4–6 months	4 weeks to > 6 months
2 Slap on the ear	62.5	4–6 weeks	4–6 weeks	3 weeks to > 6 months
3 Swimming accident	60	1–3 weeks	1–3 weeks	1 week to 3 months
4 Barotrauma	50	1–3 weeks	1–3 weeks	1 week to > 6 months
5 Instrumental cleaning of ear canal	100	1–6 weeks	4–6 weeks	< 1 week to 3 months
6 Foreign body	100	1–6 weeks	1–3 weeks	< 1 week to 3 months
7 Irrigation of ear canal	33	1–3 weeks	1–3 weeks	1–3 weeks
8 Thermal injury	66	7 weeks to 3 months	7 weeks to 3 months	7 weeks to > 6 months
9 After falling or being hit	50	4–6 weeks	4–6 weeks	1–6 weeks
10 Traffic accident	71	1–3 weeks	1–3 weeks	1 week to > 6 months
11 No detailed information available	50	7 weeks to 3 months	7 weeks to 3 months	7 weeks to 3 months

injuries caused either during attempts to clean the EEC or by foreign bodies) on the other, the optimal time periods coincided fairly well. While the underlying mechanisms are similar in the two groups, patients of categories 3 and 6 should have been more prone to superinfections than those of categories 2 and 5. The present comparison indicates either that superinfections occur less frequently than commonly thought or that they no longer play much of a role in the era of antibiotics.

Times required for spontaneous healing of some of the mechanical injuries were very short, often shorter than 1 week. For injuries caused by explosions, they were very long. This discrepancy may have been caused by the difference in the absolute size of the perforations involved. Those produced mechanically were often not larger than a myringotomy opening, whereas those caused by explosions were usually much larger. In many cases, the information about the size of the perforation was not precise enough; thus, they could not be ordered by size to answer the question just raised. Perforations after thermal traumata stand out in this respect. The time required for healing was excessively long. Since this type of injury produces actual tissue defects, this finding is not really surprising. In general, the structural repair achieved by spontaneous healing must be regarded as good. In 4 cases, however, the TM was elevated above the mallar handle, standing free of it. 2 of these cases had been caused by explosions and one each by a foreign body and a blunt head trauma. Reijnen and Kuijpers [356] saw the same type of repair in animal experiments after allowing total TM defects to regenerate.

Table XIV presents a survey of the results obtained in 381 cases of perforated TM by following various forms of active therapy.

Table XIV. Therapeutic results achieved by various measures (for explanations cf. text)

Form of therapy	Number of cases	Healed	Not healed	Lost to follow-up	Percent healed
Covering the perforation	51 (+ 7)	40	8 (+7)	3	72.7
Wound adaptation	87 (+ 7)	64	5 (+7)	18	84.2
Type I tympanoplasty	182 (+14)	140 (+10)	21 (+2)	21 (+2)	86.7
Types II and III	25	16	2	7	88.8
Multiple interventions types I–III	22	12	7	3	63.1
Total	381	282	45	54	86.2

Table XV. Therapeutic results of all tympanoplastic procedures, including multiple interventions

Tympanoplasty type	Number of surgical interventions	Healed	Not healed	Lost to follow-up	Percent healed
Type I	238	159	53	26	75
Types II and III	32	18	7	7	72

The successes achieved, as shown in the last column of table XIV and expressed as percentages, excluded those patients who did not show up for their control examinations. The numbers given in parentheses in the various columns refer to those cases in which TM covering or wound approximation had not been successful so that a tympanoplasty had to be carried out at a later time. These patients, although listed twice in each respective column, were, of course, counted only once for the determination of the success rate.

A number of repeat operations were carried out when the perforation had recurred after the first tympanoplasty. 17 patients underwent surgery twice, 5 patients 3 times. The numbers presented in table XIV give only the outcome of the final operation. However, if one does not simply consider the final outcome and counts every surgical intervention on its own, the results are less good (table XV).

When only the final results are considered (table XIV), wound approximation and the various types of tympanoplasty (including those in which the ossicular chain was repaired) achieved almost equal rates of success. Only the covering of the TM and multiple surgery produced inferior results. When, however, each tympanoplastic intervention was considered separately on its own (table XV), the results of wound approximation, as given in table XIV, were superior.

Subdivision of the therapeutic results presented in table XV according to the various causes (as given in table XIV) would have once more yielded figures much too small for a meaningful analysis. Table XVI therefore lists the number of cases treated by the various procedures in the different cause categories, but gives the rate of success (ratio healed/not healed) for each category as a whole. Patients who had not shown up for the final examination were once more excluded from this evaluation. The numbers in parentheses in several columns refer again to those cases in which tympanoplastic procedures had to be carried out, after TM covering or wound approximation had turned out to be unsuccessful.

Table XVI. Therapeutic results of different measures for various causes of trauma

Cause	Covering the perforation	Wound adaptation	Type I TP	Types II and III TP	Multipe interventions	Total number	Percent healed
1 Explosion	4 (+1)	17 (+1)	41 (+2)	5	4	73	82.8
2 Slap on the ear	25 (+3)	35 (+3)	37 (+6)	3	8	114	90.1
3 Swimming accident	5 (+1)	10	19 (+1)	—	1	36	82.2
4 Barotrauma	3	—	9	—	2	14	83.8
5 Instrumental cleaning of ear canal	5	10 (+1)	10 (+1)	—	—	26	91
6 Foreign body	4	4	11	1	2	22	81.8
7 Irrigation of ear canal	3	—	5	1	1	10	88.8
8 Thermal injury	— 1	—	13	—	1	14	85.7
9 After falling or being hit	1(+1)	9 (+1)	15 (+2)	4	1	32	92
10 Traffic accident	—	—	14	9	1	24	76.4
11 Gunshot injury	—	—	2	—	—	2	100
12 No details given	1 (+1)	2 (+1)	6 (+2)	1	1	13	81.8
13 Skull trauma (details not known)	—	—	—	1	—	1	100

Active intervention, in contrast to simply waiting for spontaneous closure, led to a difference — albeit a small one — between the results achieved in categories 2 and 5 (slaps on the ear and instrumental cleaning of the EEC) on the one hand and categories 3 and 6 (swimming accidents and foreign bodies) on the other. However, this difference can hardly be charged to bacterial contamination, since in category 7 (injuries caused by irrigation of the EEC) therapeutic results were very good, although the ears involved might also have been infected. The good results obtained after thermal trauma deserve special mention. The fact that healing was rather poor after traffic accidents might have to do with the number and severity of concomitant ME injuries and the poor general condition of these patients.

3.4.6. Therapeutic Results: Influence of the Time of Surgery
The time interval between injury and surgery could possibly influence the therapeutic results, i.e. if operated right after the injury, TM might have

a better chance to heal than after a longer waiting period. Furthermore, ME infections, recurring in the presence of persisting perforations, might, in the long run, alter the mucous membrane in such a way that the healing process could be impaired. Finally, the simple procedures, like covering the TM and wound approximation, might have merely produced good results because they were largely employed in the early stages after injury.

Table XVII presents the therapeutic results, separated for seven different time intervals between injury and surgery, but in each category together for all procedures employed. In this and tables XVIII and XIX, the numbers given are those of all interventions carried out, not those of TM repaired. Patients who did not show up for their final examination were once more excluded from the tabulation.

22 repeat procedures are included in table XVII. 17 patients were operated twice (in 9 of them, the second operation was successful; in 6, the perforations persisted; and in 2 others, results were not known); 5 patients 3 times (3 of them ultimately with good results; in 1, the perforation persisted; and in the other, results were not known). These are 49 individual interventions, and they are listed as such. In only 5 of them was the first procedure carried out before the seventh month (once during the first week, twice between the seventh week and the third month and twice between the fourth and sixth months). In the remaining 44 patients, the first procedure was carried out after the seventh month. The percentages given in the last line refer only to the outcome of the first intervention, i.e. they disregard the repeat

Table XVII. Therapeutic results of all measures: effect of the time of surgery

	Time after injury						
	<1 week	1–3 weeks	4–6 weeks	7 weeks to 3 months	4–6 months	7 months to 3 years	> 3 years
Healed	127	28	14	16	15	33	47
Not healed	18	10	2	3	5	23	24
Lost to follow-up	27	5	3	1	3	5	9
Total number of cases	172	43	19	20	23	61	80
Percent healed	87.6	73.6	87.5	84.2	75	58.9	66.2
Percent healed after first intervention	87.6	73.6	87.5	84.2	75	65.1	66.7

operations. This is perhaps the best way of looking at the results, since the execution of second or third operations indicates a failure of the first one. (At any rate, the repeat procedures would have influenced only the results of the last two columns for the reasons already given.)

Table XVII shows that the success rate was close to 88% during the first week, but also between the fourth and the sixth week. In the interim, it dropped to about 74%. This deterioration appears to be too large to be merely accidental, suggesting that, during the period between the second and the third week, the chances for healing were less favorable than before and after. If one disregards this lapse, chances for surgical success, up to the end of the third month, were about as good as immediately after the trauma, i.e. better than 80%. Thereafter, they declined gradually to 74% between the fourth and sixth months and to 65% between the seventh month and the third year. From then, the success rate did apparently not decline any further. Even when surgery was performed after very long intervals (3–50 years), the success rate kept at a steady level of 67%, i.e. it was about the same as in the period between the seventh month and the third year.

The results given in table XVII for the various time periods were subdivided according to the different therapeutic measures employed. Tables XVIII and XIX present these more detailed results. Table XVIII shows that

Table XVIII. Therapeutic results of TM coverage and wound approximation: effect of the time of surgery

Mode of therapy	Result	Time after injury, weeks		
		< 1	1–3	4–6
TM coverage,	Healed	29	6	3
total number:	Not healed	6	6	1
54 (+3)	Lost to follow-up	3	—	—
	Total	38	12	4
	Percent healed	82.8	50	75
Wound approximation	Healed	59	2	1
total number:	Not healed	9	2	1
92 (+2)	Lost to follow-up	18	—	—
	Total	86	4	2
	Percent healed	86.7	50	50

TM covering and wound approximation were rarely done after the first week; when they were done, their rates of success declined rather precipitously with time. Later, they were only occasionally attempted, one wound approximation being successfully carried out after the third month and another after the sixth month. Of three (late) attempts to cauterize the rims of the perforation and to subsequently cover the TM, only one was successful.

Tympanoplastic procedures (table XIX) were carried out over a much longer time span, i.e. as early as the day of the injury and as late as 50 years later, the very late ones being old war-related injuries caused by explosions. In table XIX, results are subdivided into two groups: (1) simple closures of TM perforations (i.e. type I tympanoplasty) and (2) those including ossicular-chain repair (i.e. type II and III tympanoplasties). In both parts of the table, the success rate is once more given twice: on top, counting only the results of the first intervention, and on the bottom, those obtained by *all* operations, including repeat procedures. 3 cases of type I tympanoplasty could not be fitted into any time period. They represent the '+3' entry on the left side.

As was pointed out already in connection with table XVII, the best way of looking at the results is to consider only those obtained after the first procedure. Moreover, the results given in the bottom half of table XIX (type II and III tympanoplasties) represent a very small number, i.e. only 32. When there are not more than 2–4 cases in a given column, success rates are statistically without any significance. Therefore, the bottom part of table XIX is reproduced here only for the sake of the record. Discussion will be limited to its top part.

Only very few procedures were carried out in the interval between the fourth and sixth week. The success rate of 100% is once more statistically not significant: one single failure would have lowered it to 90%. Nevertheless, the temporal distribution is the same as that given in table XVIII for the overall results.

The results obtained after thermal injuries and their temporal distribution need extra comments because of the suggestions made by some earlier authors, i.e. that the chances of success improve the longer one waits. The outcome of 14 operations carried out in the same number of patients is presented in table XX.

Type I tympanoplasties were carried out in all patients. One operation, 2 years after the original injury, was not successful; a type III revision three years later brought the desired result. (This 15th case is not included in table XX.)

Table XIX. Therapeutic results of tympanoplasties: effect of the time of surgery

Therapeutic measure	Result	Time after injury						
		< 1 week	1–3 weeks	4–6 weeks	7 weeks to 3 months	4–6 months	7 months to 3 years	> 3 years
Type I, total number: 213 (+3)	Healed	39	18	9	13	13	25	31
	Not healed	3	2	—	3	4	14	17
	Lost to follow-up	5	5	—	1	2	3	6
	Total	47	25	9	17	19	42	54
	Percent healed	92.8	90	100	81.3	76.5	64.1	64.6
Same, including repeated surgery (235 cases)	Percent healed	92.8	90	100	81.3	76.5	59.2	63.1
Types II and III, total number: 32	Healed	—	2	1	3	1	2	11
	Not healed	—	—	—	—	1	2	2
	Lost to follow-up	1	—	3	—	1	1	1
	Total	1	2	4	3	3	5	14
	Percent healed	—	100	100	100	50	50	84.6
Types I–III, including repeated surgery (267 cases)	Percent healed	92.8	90.9	100	84.2	73.7	58.5	67.1

Table XX. Surgical results after thermal injuries

Number	Time after injury						
	<1 week	1–3 weeks	4–6 weeks	7 weeks to 3 months	4–6 months	7 months to 3 years	>3 years
11 Healed	—	1	—	1	3	3	3
3 Not healed	1	—	—	—	—	1	1
14 Total	1	1	—	1	3	4	4

Surgical failures after thermal injuries, if they occurred, were encountered at early interventions, i.e. within the first week, as well as during later periods, i.e. beyond the seventh month. The general distribution, both with respect to time and magnitude of the success rate, was similar to that of the overall results given in table XIX for other forms of injuries.

The possibility existed that foreign bodies remaining in the ME for long periods of time might impair the chances of surgical success. In 4 of the present number of patients, foreign bodies had lodged in the ME for unknown, but presumably long, periods of time. During surgery, inflammatory reactions and granulation tissue were found. Yet, in 3 of the 4 cases TM closure was achieved on the very first attempt. It was only in the fourth case that neither the first attempt nor a second attempt was successful.

3.4.7. Therapeutic Results: Influence of Patient's Age

Some authors advise not to carry out tympanoplasties at an advanced age. Age-dependent degenerations are said to lower the chances of success. *Bocca* (cited after [349]) draws the line already at age 50, *Femenić and Subotić* [110] at age 60. Table XXI was compiled to check whether these assumptions would be valid for the management of posttraumatic TM perforations or not. Cases, separated by chronological age in decades, are presented in two groups: (1) conservative management, and (2) active, surgical intervention. In group 2 (surgical intervention), the age at the time of surgery was entered. (Hence, the age distribution of table XXI differs somewhat from that of table IX, which gave the age at the time of the injury.) The rate of success is given first for both groups in combination and secondly for the operated ears only. In this type of statistic, repeat procedures cannot be considered. Only the final result achieved was therefore entered for each patient.

If one takes a look at the total success rate regardless of the type of

Table XXI. 531 eardrum perforations: therapeutic results — effect of patient's age

	Age in decades, years							
	0–10	11–20	21–30	31–40	41–50	51–60	61–70	71–80
1 Conservative management								
Healed	12	12	18	9	4	5	2	—
Not healed	8	12	22	13	15	10	5	3
2 Surgical management								
Healed	21	49	84	56	44	16	10	2
Not healed	2	5	14	9	7	6	2	—
Lost to follow-up	3	9	19	11	7	1	3	1
Total	46	87	157	98	77	38	22	6
Percent healed of the total	76.7	78.2	73.9	74.7	68.5	56.7	63.1	40
Percent healed of surgical cases only	91.3	90.7	85.7	86.1	86.2	72.7	83.3	100

management, one could indeed gain the impression that the chances of success might decrease with age. However, if one limits consideration to the cases that were treated actively, one will find that the success rate stayed approximately constant with age at levels of 83–91%. There was only one exception from this rule, the group 51–60 years of age (72.7%). In the group from 71 to 80 years, results are statistically meaningless on account of the small number of cases. The decrease of the percentage figures of total healing with advancing age might be accounted for by the fact that a relatively large proportion of older patients refused surgery.

3.4.8. Therapeutic Results: Influence of the Degree of Mastoid Pneumatization

The frequency of occurrence of chronic otitis media of the mucopurulent type is known to correlate with the degree of pneumatization in an inverse manner. That is to say, chronic otitis occurs more frequently in ears, in which pneumatization is poor [71, 72]. A low degree of pneumatization is thought to be related to constitutional factors [385]. These might also affect the healing of posttraumatic TM perforations. In the present series, therefore, the relative degree of mastoid pneumatization was assessed by planimetric means in all patients with TM perforations, provided a Schüller X-ray picture had been taken during the course of their clinical treatment. (The procedure was described above in chapter 2.3.1.)

X-Ray pictures of 270 patients with TM ruptures could be evaluated. In 183 of them, the perforations had either healed on their own or after appropriate active measures (group A). In the remaining 87 patients, they had not healed (group B). In both groups, the degree of pneumatization showed a wide distribution (fig. 1), i.e. from 1.0 cm² to 23.0 cm² for group A and from 1.0 cm² to 21.0 cm² for group B; however, the two maxima were clearly separated. The average pneumatization index for group A was 8.91 cm² and for group B 4.7 cm². In spite of the considerable variation of individual values in both groups, the statistical difference turned out to be highly significant: contingency tables indicated a χ^2 value of 29.179, corresponding to a p of 0.0003. The significance is thus clearly beyond the 0.1% limit of probable errors, and the correlation between the degree of mastoid pneumatization and the tendency for self-repair appears to be positive.

3.4.9. Audiometric Results: Influence of the Mode of Therapy Employed

Evaluation of postsurgical audiometric results should be limited to those patients in whom the perforations were successfully closed; but that can only

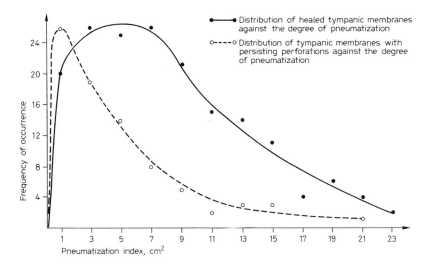

Fig. 1. Tympanic membrane perforations: the effect of pneumatization on its healing. Both curves are fitted by inspection. The degree of pneumatization is expressed in terms of the pneumatization index in cm² (cf. chapter 2.3.1).

be done, if pre- and postsurgical audiograms are available. The first criterion applied to 344 patients, but the second one to only 200. To avoid the difficulties of small samples once more, only the average audiometric gain for five frequencies (0.25, 1, 2, 4, and 8 kHz) was determined for five different categories of therapy. The results are presented in table XXII. This table includes 4 patients, in whom type I tympanoplasties had failed to produce any auditory improvements, 1 in whom hearing had further deteriorated by 5 dB, in spite of multiple surgery, and 2 more, in whom, after type I tympanoplasty, it had deteriorated by 10 dB. In 5 patients, the average audiometric gain was better than 30 dB (4 type I tympanoplasties and 1 wound approximation).

Table XXII indicates that in the cases examined closure of the perforation had improved ME sound conduction nominally by 13.4 ± 7.5 dB. Standard deviations were relatively large, due to the aberrant results in the groups with small numbers (i.e. groups 1, 2 and 5).

(There is one flaw in such an assessment and that concerns the measurement of presurgical thresholds in the presence of TM perforations, as in the present cases. When one employs precalibrated earphones, TM perforations

Table XXII. Audiometric results: effect of the mode of therapy

Therapeutic mode	Number of cases	Conductive gain, dB	1 SD, dB
1 Spontaneous healing	22	16.3	± 4.3
2 Eardrum coverage	15	11.3	± 7.7
3 Wound adaptation	46	13.1	± 5.8
4 Tympanoplasty	109	13.1	± 7.9
5 Multiple surgery	8	14.1	± 8.6
Total	200	13.4	± 7.2

lower the sound pressure levels in the EEC, especially at low frequencies, i.e. the readings obtained are worse than what they should be. The error may be as large as 10–15 dB [490].)

Differences among groups and deviations from the average value of the total (line 6) were statistically not significant. Under some simplifying assumptions, table XXII suggests that closure of the perforation produces approximately the same audiometric gain — regardless of the mode of therapy chosen.

3.4.10. Audiometric Results: Influence of the Time Interval between Trauma and the Onset of Therapy

Audiograms taken after a considerable lapse of time after surgery were available in 221 patients; the ruptured TM had healed under various forms of management. The average hearing losses still existing were determined under the rules given in the previous chapter (chapter 3.4.6). Results, presented in figure 2, are given as functions of the time interval between trauma and the onset of therapy, without regard to presurgical hearing levels. The time intervals were made larger than those chosen for the evaluation of the structural results given in table XIX (chapter 3.4.5); otherwise, the numbers per interval would have become too small for statistical purposes. (Multiple interventions are entered into an extra column.) In each column, results are grouped in five different classes, depending on the severity of the remaining hearing losses.

Figure 2 indicates that the percentage of persisting hearing losses, larger than 10 dB, increased with the length of the time interval, while, simultaneously, that of small losses, between 0 and 10 dB, decreased.

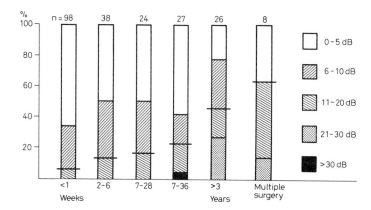

Fig. 2. Tympanic membrane perforations: Conductive loss components (in decibels) remaining after surgical repair for various time intervals between injury and surgery (n = 221). Values are given in percent for each time interval. The heavy line in each time column delineates the losses > 10 dB.

Postsurgical hearing losses, larger than 20 dB, are found in figure 2 under two conditions only: either when the time interval was longer than 6 months or following multiple interventions. Hence, the functional results were indeed affected by the time interval between trauma and the onset of therapy.

3.5. Discussion of Clinical and Roentgenological Results and of the Postmortem Findings

It will be recalled that more than one half of all TM ruptures were caused by blast trauma. Direct, mechanical injuries as well as those associated with blunt head trauma contributed only 15.5% each. Traffic accidents, an important factor in general accident statistics, produced a mere 7%. There was only 1 case of a TM ruptured during a barotrauma, an observation that is in line with previous findings [241]. Since pressure differentials become generally larger under water, ruptured TM were seen more often in divers, i.e. 21 times.

It was in only 1 patient that a perforation was suspected as having been produced during an attempted extraction of a foreign body from the EEC.

The rarity of this type of injury is probably a direct consequence of the many warnings issued against such attempts [221, 239, 313, 397]. On the other hand, the relatively large number of iatrogenic TM perforations produced while EEC were being irrigated should give rise to some thought. Whereas the warnings against instrumental cleaning of the EEC are being heeded to some extent, it appears that the danger arising from merely irrigating the EEC, unless done by trained hands, is grossly underestimated. That mechanical cleaning done by the patient himself is potentially quite dangerous is illustrated by the large number of TM perforations, i.e. 37, produced in this manner.

Ruptures were most frequently found in the anteroinferior quadrant, regardless of the mode of injury. However, to assume therefore that the underlying mechanism should be the same in all instances cannot be correct. The cadaver experiments of *Zaufal* [475–477] and of *Passow* [339] provided good explanations for the way perforations are produced mechanically. As already mentioned, these authors observed that instruments introduced into the EEC slide off the posterosuperior wall so that they eventually impinge on the anteroinferior quadrant. With respect to injuries produced during welding operations, the observation of *Möbius* [304], i.e. that, as a rule, the walls of the EEC remain untouched, was confirmed. This fact may be explained by the protection provided by the ceruminal cover of the canal skin [168, 371, 446]. Discussion of the mode of origin of TM injuries produced by blast trauma will be postponed until after the description of pertinent experimental studies in chapter 3.6.

Marginal TM ruptures in the posterosuperior quadrant, although rare, occur typically in conjunction with longitudinal TB fractures produced by blunt head trauma. In the present material, they were diagnosed with certainty in only 4 clinical patients, out of a total of 79 such traumata seen. In the postmortem material, there were 5 cases of longitudinal fractures, in which the roofs of the EEC were shattered, accompanied by extensive destructions of the skull basis and the squama, i.e. by injuries that would have been hardly compatible with the survival of the patient. Yet, there were only 2 marginal TM perforations in the total group, compared to 11 intact TM.

Among clinical patients with longitudinal TB fractures caused by blunt head trauma, as well as in the corresponding postmortem specimens, central perforations were much more in evidence than marginal perforations. Most of them were located in the anteroinferior quadrant. One or the other might have been produced by a fall on the ear, i.e. they could have actually been the result of a blast trauma. However, this was definitely not true in the postmortem cases. In all of them the site of the impact was found at some distance away from the ear.

All of these central perforations were located in the middle of the pars tensa and not in the region of the annulus. This finding contradicts the notion of *Corradi* [63, 64], i.e. that the mechanical vibration might lead to a separation of bone and soft tissues. On the other hand, a good case can be made for *Passow's* [339] concept of 1905. He thought that a skull trauma might produce a transient deformation of the tympanic annulus, with a subsequent (elastic) return to its normal configuration. The TM, tensed by the deformation of its osseous frame, might thus be overstressed and rupture.

Böhm [36] used the term *'Berstungsruptur'* (bursting rupture) of the TM to characterize this type of injury. He argued that the osseous frame when compressed along one axis should expand along the axis lying normal to it, thus overstretching parts of the TM. This notion was endorsed by *Imhofer* [209]. (Such a mechanism might also be responsible for the infraction of the floor of the EEC.) An analysis of the present postmortem material showed that, when the elastic limits of the tympanic annulus were exceeded, it was usually fractured in its posterosuperior region and sometimes also in the anteroinferior one. This finding suggested that the almost circular annulus is being elliptically deformed with its long axis in the sagittal plane, stretching the TM in the same direction. This suggestion is supported by an observation of *Guerrier* et al. [160], i.e. that it is especially the tympanic annulus that is being deformed when the temporal bone is subjected to a sudden impact. The same authors were able to demonstrate with the aid of photoelastic techniques that a blunt trauma to the lateral base of the skull forces the tympanic roof downward and the lateral attic wall sideways, thus increasing the distance between the posterosuperior and the anteroinferior portions of the tympanic annulus. Such osseous deformations might well stretch the TM beyond its limits. This line of reasoning rests on the assumption that the elastic limits of the TM and of its osseous frame are of the same order of magnitude, since blunt skull traumata are known to lead to separate injuries of either structure alone as well as to combined injuries.

With respect to the therapy employed, one should not only look at the factors that evidently promoted healing, but also at those that did not play a role in this regard, although they were thought to do so at one time or another. The different modes of injury, for example, did not affect healing (cf. table XVI). It might be recalled that neither the rates of success nor the times required for complete healing differed significantly between causes that are thought to invite infections (swimming accidents, irrigation of the EEC or foreign bodies lodged in the ear) and those that are less likely to do so (mechanical cleaning of the EEC, blows to the ear). Nevertheless, *Korkis* [255] in 1946, saw healing still being delayed whenever a TM rupture had been followed by an ME infection. That this is no longer true may have to do with the early onset of surgical treatment combined with the administration of antibiotics. This type of management gave good results even in cases of chronic infections caused by, and maintained by, foreign bodies that had remained in the ME for extended periods of time (3 out of 4 cases.) Even after thermal injuries, healing occurred in substantially the same manner as was determined for the average of the total group. Spontaneous healing (in 14% of cases) was even better, if only slightly, than that seen for the whole group (11.5%). The rate of success after surgical management was also quite satisfactory, i.e. 85%. These results were considerably better than those obtained by others (38% [133]; 63% [151]; 63% [288]) and even better than those of *Vick* [446]. Hence, the chances of success of tympanoplastic procedures in cases of thermal injury were about as good as in those produced by other modes of injury.

Age also had minimal effects on healing. For reasons already discussed (cf. chapter 3.4.7), the relative frequency of surgery decreased after the 50th year of life, thus necessarily increasing the percentage of persisting perforations. Yet, the surgical success rate remained rather constant in patients that did undergo surgery. This observation is supported by the histological findings of *Fleischer* [117], who was unable to demonstrate any morphological alterations in the ME of older people attributable to age. In turn, it corroborates *Plester*'s [349] clinical impression, i.e. that the chances of the TM to heal do not decrease with advancing age; hence, that there is no age limit for tympanoplasty.

It was rather striking that active interventions of all kinds gave much better results than conservative measures. In the age of microsurgery, therefore, the old wait-and-see attitude — rightfully called 'watchful neglect' [13] — should be considered obsolete. Among the various forms of therapy, type I tympanoplasty and wound approximation produced approximately the same rate of success, i.e. 86.7 and 84.2%, respectively, whereas merely covering the perforation was somewhat less effective with only 72.7%. This almost uniform efficacy of the various surgical measures should not make one overlook the importance of two other factors that help significantly to influence the decision criteria pro and con the various forms of surgical interventions.

The first of these factors concerns the size and kind of the perforation. That is to say, mere coverage of a perforation should only be considered when it is small and when the wound edges are properly facing one another. However, when the edges are torn and rolled up, when tissue defects exist or when there is any suspicion that the ossicular chain might be damaged, tympanoplasty is the method of choice. These criteria imply that, by definition, tympanoplasty is indicated under the least favorable conditions; but its rate of success is still the best. With respect to the mere covering of a perforation, both points apply in a reverse manner.

The second factor arises from the fact that covering the perforation or approximating the wound margins were rarely, if ever, done when traumatic ruptures were older than 1 week. If done late, their rates of success were definitely inferior. Hence, these two methods required decisions that were selective in the time domain. Admittedly, however, tympanoplastic procedures also produced poorer results when the intervention was delayed; the success rate became poor from the structural standpoint and from the functional one as well. That is to say, even though perforations might have been effectively closed, the percentage of poor audiometric results kept continuously increasing with time, beginning with the second week after injury. Early active intervention, if at all possible during the first week, is therefore desirable for good structural as well as functional results. One ought to forgo simpler measures, such as covering the TM, in favor of the more thorough ones, wound approximation or tympanoplasty, because of their superior result. However, the present series does not permit to decide whether this strategy should also be adopted with respect to thermal injuries or whether one should follow the recommendations of others [e.g. 133, 151], i.e. to delay surgery for at least 6 months. And then again, 5 of the eleven good results in the present series had resulted from surgery performed between the second week and the sixth month. Hence, one may only state that early surgery did at least do as well as late intervention.

As regards the time of intervention and the kind of surgery to be used, the surgeon has a rather free choice. However, two other factors determining the outcome are out of his control: first, the general condition of the patient (this was shown by the fact that, with traffic accidents, the success rate, 76%, was clearly less than the average because of concomitant, severe injuries to other parts of the body); secondly, the pneumatization of the mastoid (good pneumatization had been found to improve the chances of success). Nevertheless, it must be mentioned in this respect that, although the degree of pneumatization is thought to reflect the potency of the ME *mucosa* [385], the healing of a TM perforation is clearly promoted by the action of its *epithelial* layer [281, 355, 356, 367]. One must conclude therefore that the healing of TM perforations depends on the condition of the ME mucosa in a manner that is not properly understood at this time.

3.6. Blast Injury of the Tympanic Membrane: Our Observations

During the course of an explosion, the air pressure changes with time in a biphasic manner. Measurements at a stationary point near the source register first a positive, sharp pressure peak of short duration: 1.5 msec [232] and up to 6–7 msec [105]. This is followed by a negative phase of a lesser peak pressure, but of longer duration (fig. 3). When such an event spreads from its source in all directions, it loses amplitude in proportion to the square of the distance; but it gains in duration, which means it loses high-frequency components. Witness the sharp and brief crack produced by a nearby thunderclap and compare it to the dull, rumbling quality of thunder originating farther away. Pulses are *'smeared out in time'*. This *low-pass filtering* is a general property of most transmission systems, including free air [435].

The notion [81, 164] that TM might rupture under the effect of the negative pressure phase is not very probable. The positive pressure peak is invariably higher in amplitude than the negative one (cf. fig. 3). This is at least partly due to the fact that the limiting value of the negative pressure is 0 mm Hg since the resting pressure, the normal atmospheric pressure, is 760 mm Hg. Most TM are capable of withstanding a differential of 760 mm Hg [473]. Most likely, therefore, if a TM ruptures, it yields to the positive pressure wave that displaces it inward. (This point will be further discussed in chapter 3.6.3.)

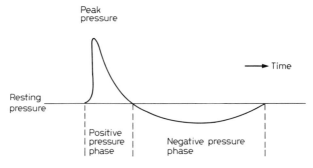

Fig. 3. Typical time course of the pressure change during and after an explosion (adapted from [232]).

Many authors believe that an explosive impulse should rupture predominantly the TM of the ear that is facing the source of the explosion and would thus be directly exposed to the blast [255, 402, 478]. Explosions occurring in enclosed spaces are considered the exception, since the pressure pulse undergoes multiple reflections and diffractions [232, 433]. Long-duration (i.e. low-frequency) impulses should reach both ears with about the same intensity, since they are subject to strong diffractions [374].

Schwartze and Eysell [384], and *Eysell* [106] later on on his own, were able to show experimentally that a membrane covering an air-filled, but otherwise closed and hard-walled, cylinder of large volume could be ruptured by relatively small impulses. An identical membrane covering a cylinder of smaller volume proved to be more resistant.

Eysell [106] applying this model concept to the human ear, expressed the opinion that air pressure impulses of a given magnitude and quality should rupture the TM more easily when the pneumatization is extensive than when it is poor. This notion was recently adopted by other authors [70, 119] with respect to the mechanism of barotrauma.

The above experimental results had to be expected on the basis of general physical laws. The situation is schematically depicted in figure 4. Under the conditions cited, the cylinder encloses a given air volume V; the pressure p within shall be equal to the resting pressure in the environment, say 760 mm Hg. When the membrane closing off one of its sides is subjected to an increase in the environmental air pressure p, it is displaced into the cylinder, the volume displacement being ΔV. The air in the cylinder is compressed in the amount of $V' = V - \Delta V$ and the pressure is increased to the level of $p' = p + \Delta p$. The displacement of the membrane ceases as soon as an

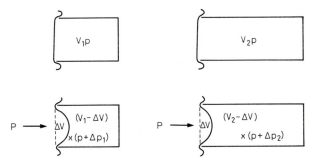

Fig. 4. Pressure and volume changes in short (left) and long (right) cylinders (schematic). $V_1 < V_2$; $V \cdot p = \text{const.}$; $P = E + \Delta p$.

equilibrium is established beween the increased environmental pressure P and the opposing forces, the sum of the elastic restoring force of the membrane (E) and that due to the pressure increment in the cylinder, Δp, i.e.

$$P = E + \Delta p. \tag{1}$$

Since the restoring force of the membrane remains proportional to the volume change, ΔV, i.e. as long as the relation is linear, this equation may be simplified to read:

$$p' \sim \Delta p. \tag{2}$$

For a constant and given ΔV.
According to the law of Boyle and Mariotte,

$$p \times V = constant, \tag{3}$$

again as long as the system behaves linearly. Therefore, when the pressure is increased,

$$p' \times V' = (p + \Delta p)(V - \Delta V), \tag{4}$$

which may be rewritten as

$$p + \Delta p = \frac{p' \times V'}{V - \Delta V}. \tag{5}$$

Consequently,

$$\Delta p = \frac{p' \times V'}{V - \Delta V} - p. \tag{6}$$

For various values of V, the relation $p' \times V'$ is given as a family of hyperbolas. With increasing V, these are being displaced to the right (fig. 5). Assuming a constant volume displacement ΔV, e.g. the ΔV which is needed for a membrane rupture, one finds, according to equation 6, that Δp must be *relatively large*, when $V \geqq \Delta V$ (curve labeled V_1 in fig. 5), and *relatively small*, when $V \gg \Delta V$ (curve labeled V_2 in fig. 5).

3.6.1. Our Clinical Findings

The present series comprised 110 TM ruptured by explosions, including 25 bilateral ruptures. This group was suitable for testing the first of the above hypotheses, i.e. the notion that the ear facing the source of an explosion is more likely to be ruptured than the other (table XXIII).

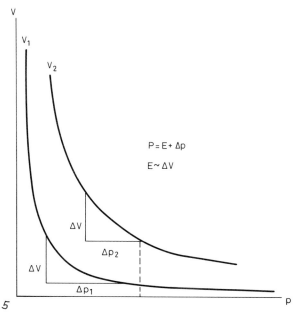

Fig. 5. Static pressure-volume characteristic for two air volumes ($V_1 < V_2$). Equal volume changes, ΔV, produce different pressure changes, Δp_1 and Δp_2.

Table XXIII. TM ruptures, unilateral and bilateral, produced by various types of explosions

Type of explosion	Unilateral ruptures	bilateral ruptures
Land mine	3	5
Artillery shell	7	1
Hand grenade	1	1
Blasting	—	3
Noise maker	12	—
Handgun	4	—
Toy balloon	2	8

The way the head had been held relative to the site of the explosion could of course no longer be ascertained. Yet, a number of different kinds of explosions had produced unilateral as well as bilateral TM ruptures, an observation that cast some doubt on the above notion.

Table XXIII shows that unilateral ruptures were caused especially by explosions of low power (noise makers and handguns). This is a logical finding: such devices produce injuries only when detonated near the ear. Consequently, there is a pronounced head-shadow effect so that the pressure acting on the opposite ear should, as a rule, be too small to do much harm. Explosions of higher power, on the other hand, are seen to produce bilateral TM ruptures more frequently. They are capable of acting at larger distances. And in a wider, and therefore more diffuse, field the head shadow is no longer effective. That is to say, the position of the head relative to the source does no longer matter. These considerations are supported by earlier findings on 187 war-wounded patients [433].

There is another factor that must be mentioned in this connection: when the angle of incidence of a sound coming into the EEC is changed by 90°, i.e. from direct to grazing incidence, the loss of sound pressure at the TM is a mere 5 dB at all frequencies save those above 6 kHz. This equalizing effect is mainly brought about by the pinna that funnels sound rather effectively into the EEC [499].

In table XXIII, the injuries produced by detonations of toy balloons filled with hydrogen were placed in a separate category. Admittedly, these detonations are of low power. Yet, 8 of the 10 TM ruptures observed were bilateral ones; 4 of them had occurred in enclosed spaces. Therefore, they had to be handled separately. The findings made are in agreement with those of *Kerr* [232] and *Langenbeck* [263] that were already mentioned.

3.6.2. Planimetric Assessments

The hypothesis of *Schwartze and Eysell* [384] was tested by assessing the extent of mastoid pneumatization in the ears of patients with unilateral perforations and of those with bilateral perforations.

In 22 patients with unilateral TM ruptures caused by explosions, pneumatization indices were determined for the injured ears as well as for the uninjured ones (for method cf. chapter 2.3.1). The distribution of the results is given in figure 6. The mean pneumatization index of the uninjured ears was 10.83 cm^2 and of the injured ears 5.95 cm^2. In a paired-comparison t-test, these two values differed significantly from each other (t = 4.04; p < 0.001).

With the exception of 5 patients, the lesion had always occurred on the side of the *lesser* pneumatization. In 4 of the 5 exceptions, the difference between the two sides was less than 1.0 cm^2 (the average difference in the total series being 4.88 cm^2). That is, in these cases the degree of pneumatization was about equal on the two sides. These results contradict the earlier notions of *Eysell*: The more vulnerable ear was the one with the *lesser* pneumatization, not the one with the *more extensive* pneumatization. That is to say, TM ruptures produced by explosions were *inversely* correlated with the degree of pneumatization. The occurrence of ruptures did not appear to be related to the fact whether the involved ear had faced, or not faced, the site of the explosion.

To check this notion further, pneumatization indices were determined in 13 patients with bilateral TM ruptures produced by explosions. Of every pair, the ear with the higher degree of pneumatization was put in group 1, that with the lesser degree in group 2. For the first group, the mean value was 8.95 cm^2 and for the second group 6.87 cm^2. The average difference between the two sides, 2.08 cm^2, was significantly smaller than that found in cases with unilateral lesions (t = 2.09; 0.05 > p > 0.01).

These results suggest that, if the degree of pneumatization differs significantly between the two sides, unilateral TM ruptures are likely to occur, taking place on the side of the *lesser* pneumatization. Otherwise, i.e. when the degree of pneumatization on the two sides is approximately equal, ruptures are more likely to occur simultaneously on both sides.

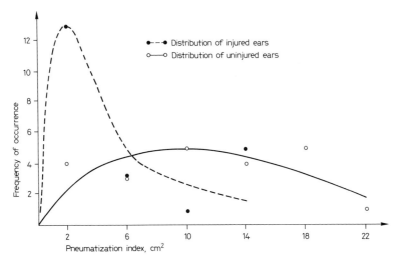

Fig. 6. Distribution of pneumatization in a group of ears injured by explosions and in another group not injured.

To examine the question whether or not ears with relatively small degrees of pneumatization might be less resistant even to slowly occurring atmospheric pressure changes, ears damaged by barotraumata were also evaluated planimetrically. On the injured side, the mean pneumatization index was 7.5 cm^2; on the uninjured side it was 10.05 cm^2. A paired-comparison t-test showed that the difference was statistically significant (t = 3.02; $0.001 < p < 0.01$).

On first sight, this result may seem to indicate that ears with relatively small degrees of pneumatization might possess TM with a relatively small resistance to air pressure differentials across them; this could perhaps be related to the early childhood infections that are held to be responsible for the impairment in pneumatization in the first place. However, it turned out that in cases of barotrauma the frequency of injury on the side of the lesser degree of pneumatization was only slightly and statistically insignificantly higher than on the other side (ratio = 0.65; p = 0.13), a finding that was in clear contrast to lesions caused by explosions (ratio = 0.777; p = 0.0085). Thus, the explanation cannot be that simple.

Table XXIV summarizes once more the pneumatization indices for the injuries produced by the two pressure-related causes. An explanation for the findings just described will be offered in chapter 3.6.3.3, following the discussion of our own experimental results.

Table XXIV. Degree of mastoid pneumatization of ears injured by explosions and barotraumata: paired comparison

Type of trauma	Mean pneumatization index of the ears without trauma (1,3) or with more extensive pneumat.(2), cm^2	Mean pneumatization index of the ears with trauma (1,3) or with less extensive pneumat.(2), cm^2	Probability of significant difference (p)
(1) Unilateral injury	10.83 ± 5.84	5.95 ± 4.90	0.01 > p > 0.001
(2) Bilateral injury	8.95 ± 4.87	6.87 ± 4.57	p > 0.05
(3) Barotrauma	10.05 ± 4.16	7.50 ± 4.78	p > 0.05
Explosions: difference in paired comparisons	unilateral injury	bilateral injury	probability
	4.88 ± 5.66	2.08 ± 1.80	0.05 > p > 0.01

3.6.3. Our Experimental Studies

In an effort to clear up some of the disputed points further, experiments were conducted in human cadaver ears, removed as soon as possible after death.

3.6.3.1. Materials and Methods

(1) The volume of the total ME spaces has been repeatedly measured: 0–25 ml [122]; 2–22 ml [308]; 6–22 ml [396]. It was of interest to learn how these volumes might be distributed into the ME proper and the mastoid spaces. It was therefore decided to measure the volume of ME and antrum, on which only estimates exist, e.g. approximately 2 ml [125].

The ME volume was determined on 8 ears. The dura was separated from the upper surface of the petrous pyramid and, with the aid of a drill, the roof of ME and antrum removed under microscopic control. The tympanal orifice of the Eustachian tube was sealed off with dental cement and so were the retrotympanal spaces beyond the antrum. ME and antrum were then filled with water exactly up to the level of the roof. (Some detergent added to the water prevented formation of air bubbles, and the addition of indigocarmine let one detect leakages if and when they occurred.) In each specimen, measurements were repeated 5 times. The final result was their arithmetic average.

(2) The pressure-volume characteristic of the TM (wich should eventually become nonlinear) was determined in 6 specimens. A preparation, consisting only of the tympanic annulus and the TM with the malleus attached, was securely fastened in a device that permitted one to connect an air pressure pump on the meatal side and a graduated pipette, filled with water, on the tympanic side (fig. 7). All seals were made airtight. The pressure produced by the pump was monitored with the aid of a Statham element and a bridge system, as used for the registration of blood pressure. The resulting volume displacement of the TM was read in terms of the displacement of the fluid column.

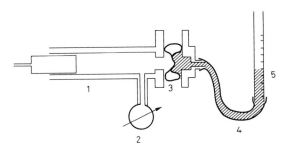

Fig. 7. Instrumental arrangement for the measurement of the static pressure-volume characteristic of human tympanic membranes (for further details cf. text). 1 = Air pressure pump; 2 = pressure-measuring bridge; 3 = tympanic membrane; 4 = connecting tube; 5 = graduated pipette.

Before each measurement, the level in the pipette was always adjusted so that no hydrostatic pressure was acting on the TM, which would have affected the measured result (cf. fig. 7). Pressure was altered in steps. Each time, after a given pressure-volume pair had been assessed, the pressure was restored to zero to check if the fluid column would return to its original level, enabling the experimenter to recognize leaks in the system if and when they had occurred. Pressure was increased up to the point at which either leakage occurred or the TM ruptured.

(3) Four preparations served to analyze the changes the TM underwent when exposed to a sudden burst of air pressure. Specimens were prepared and mounted as before, but in such a manner that the entire surface of the TM could be visualized. It was brightly illuminated by cold light. The piston of the air pump was suddenly advanced by means of a spring, the rapid pressure increase eventually rupturing the TM. Simultaneously with the pressure pulse, a high-speed movie of the TM was taken (NCA 16 HD revolving-prism camera, 3,000 frames/sec; VNF 7250 film). When viewing the movie at normal projection speeds, the experimenter was able to observe the gradual development of the TM rupture.

3.6.3.2. Experimental Results

(1) Table XXV presents the results of the volume measurements of ME and antrum. From these results and from those cited above on the total volume of the ME spaces, figure 8 was prepared. It gives the distribution of the total volume into the various subspaces.

Table XXV. ME volumes of 8 human cadaver ears

0.53 ± 0.02 ml	0.59 ± 0.03 ml
0.40 ± 0.05 ml	0.50 ± 0.02 ml
0.36 ± 0.04 ml	0.58 ± 0.03 ml
0.58 ± 0.01 ml	0.69 ± 0.02 ml

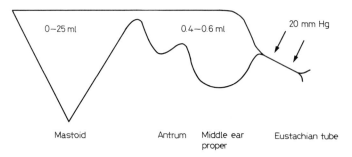

Fig. 8. Volumes of the various middle-ear spaces (schematic).

(2) The pressure-volume characteristics of 6 TM are listed in table XXVI. 4 of these cases were selected for graphical presentation. Figure 9 shows that, in spite of their individual differences, all curves are members of the same family. Near their point of origin the curves rise quite steeply to become noticeably less steep at a Δp of about 50 mm Hg. Beyond approximately 100 mm Hg, the slopes are rather small. The pressure-volume characteristic is indeed highly nonlinear over the range of measurements.

(3) In 1 of the 4 specimens, in which TM ruptures were recorded, the membrane ruptured too early for a reliable analysis. In the 3 remaining cases, the sequential pattern was identical: first, the mallar handle moved inward, displacement being maximal at the umbo. At the same time, the curved surface of the TM flattened out, especially in its lower portion. Thereafter, a shallow, inwardly directed bulge appeared in the posteroinferior quadrant, but it was of lesser magnitude than the original inward displacement. Finally, the membrane tore in a star-shaped pattern, starting near the apex of the inwardly displaced section. The torn edges first floated freely in the air stream, finally folding under on the tympanic side of the TM.

Table XXVI. Pressure-volume characteristics of six tympanic membranes. Increments in external-canal pressure (Δp) in mm Hg. Resulting volume displacements of the tympanic membrane (ΔV) in μl

Δp	Membrane No.					
	1	2	3	4	5	6
2	4	6				
4		14				
6	20	20				6
8		30		4		
10	27	30	10	4	2	15
20	32	35	17	6	4	18
30	36	42	22	7	5	20
40	39	47	27	10	5	
50	42	49	30		6	
60	45	50	32	11		20
100	47	55	35	13	8	22
150	50		36	15	9	
200			40	18	12	28
250			44		13	
300			44	20	14	
600			ruptured	24	20	

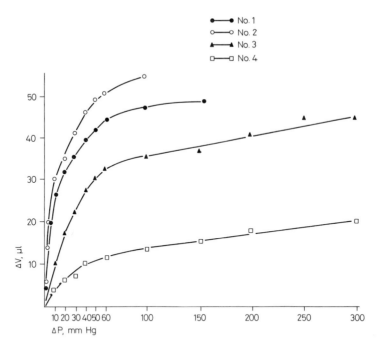

Fig. 9. Static pressure-volume displacement characteristic of four human tympanic membranes.

3.6.3.3. Discussion of Experimental Results

The lowest pressure increment, at which the volume changes were measured, was 2 mm Hg (cf. table XXVI). This corresponds approximately to an SPL of 120 dB. That is to say, most results presented in table XXVI and in figure 9 were obtained at levels considerably above the auditory range. However, if the curves of figure 9 were extrapolated toward much lower values, well within the auditory range, they would be virtually undistinguishable from linear functions.

Kobrak [489] measured the rotation of the mallar handle in a fresh human cadaver specimen over a pressure range from – 6 mm Hg (outward displacement) to + 4 mm Hg (inward displacement). On outward displacements, nonlinearity became evident at about – 5 mm Hg, but on inward displacements, already at + 1 mm Hg. The asymmetry thus demonstrated must lead to odd harmonic distortion, which has indeed been demonstrated psychophysically: The third harmonic, the first odd one, appears at about

100 dB SPL, somewhat varying with frequency [483, 491]. Hence, the width of the linear range of the TM is quite large, which, according to *Helmholtz* [486], is due to the particular shape of the membrane. As *Helmholtz* pointed out, the smallest displacements in the center of a *flat* membrane, fastened at its rim, represent already a nonlinear step. However, with a membrane that is shaped like an exponential cone and is also fastened at its rim, such as the TM, there is an initial linear range of considerable width. Eventually, of course, the displacements of such a membrane also become nonlinear as is seen in figure 9.

The high-speed motion pictures first showed a rapid inward displacement of the TM that was facilitated by a flattening out of the normally curved TM surface. This was followed by a shallow inward displacement in a restricted region. The entire event took place mainly in the inferior portion of the TM. The complexity of the displacements indicates that the membrane must undergo considerable *stretching*, the main stress occurring in the inferior region of the TM. It was in this stretched portion that the membrane eventually ruptured.

Dancer et al. [482], with the aid of holography, recorded a sequence of displacement patterns of the TM in response to air pressure pulses, 200 μs in duration. The ME was kept intact. By and large, their results were very similar to those obtained by the present method, but authors were able to carry out a *numerical* analysis. They showed that the maximal displacement of the membrane, which took place in the *anteroinferior* quadrant, increased with time at a much faster rate than that of the umbo, becoming eventually, i.e. 40 μs after the onset of the pulse, 7 times higher. For the sake of comparison, when a human TM is exposed to a steady-state sound of physiological magnitude, the ratio between maximal-membrane and umbo displacements is only 3 to 1 [497]. This once more reveals the considerable (nonlinear) stretching of the TM under the effect of an air pressure pulse.

For reasons of their experimental design, *Dancer* et al. [482] deliberately did not raise the pressure high enough to rupture the TM. However, their results strongly suggest that ruptures would have occurred in the *anteroinferior* quadrant, the site typically found in clinical patients. In the present experiments, as will be recalled, ruptures took place in the *posteroinferior* quadrant. If one regards only the ME volume (about 0.5 ml) under an ambient pressure of 760 mmHg, in inward movement of the TM of $\Delta V = 20 \mu l$ would be sufficient to raise the ME pressure by more than 20 mmHg and thus to force open the Eustachian tube. As table XXVI shows, this ΔV can be caused by a small Δp in the EEC. So a possible explanation might be, that in the posterior part of the TM its inward movement is damped by the effect of the mastoid cells, whereas in its anterior portion this damping effect is lacking because of the opening of the Eustachian tube. This could explain the observation, that most of the TM ruptured in the region of the tympanic tubal orifice, and that a good pneumatization had a protective effect against blast-induced ruptures. On the other hand, the difference may lie in the following: With the ME intact and in response to fast pulses, the impedance of the posteroinferior quadrant that lies rather closely over the promontory should be somewhat higher than that of the anteroinferior quadrant that lies over the entrance to the Eustachian tube, where the ME is much wider. Consequently, the displacements of the anteroinferior quadrant may become larger than those of the posteroinferior quadrant, inviting ruptures to take place here.

Summarizing this discussion, we may state that the TM is ruptured when being overstretched. This is brought about by abnormally large (nonlinear) displacements over a limited region, specifically in the anteroinferior quadrant.

One question that remains to be discussed is whether the Eustachian tube would be forced open by the increase in ME pressure, i.e. whether under these conditions the ME represents a completely closed system or an open one. The numerical results of *Dancer* et al. [482] suggest that the event occurs so fast that there is virtually no time to force the tube open.

We are now in a position to answer two questions that were raised earlier: (1) Why was the suggestion of *Schwartze and Eysell* [384] not correct, i.e. that a TM of an ear with a poorly pneumatized mastoid would rupture less easily than one of an ear with a well-pneumatized mastoid? (2) Why is the 'flaccid' Shrapnell's membrane rarely, if ever, ruptured?

(1) The displacements of the TM are chiefly controlled by frictional resistance, which is mainly given by that of the air being forced into, and pulled out of, the mastoid air cells when the TM is being displaced. When there is a large number of air cells, i.e. the mastoid is well-pneumatized, friction is large and TM displacements relatively small. When there is one solitary cavity, i.e. the mastoid is poorly pneumatized, friction is small and TM displacements comparatively large. Other things being equal, therefore, the TM of an ear with a poorly pneumatized mastoid is more likely to be ruptured than one of an ear with a well-pneumatized mastoid. The degree of damping varies of course with the rate of the pressure change, which in cases of barotrauma is generally slower than in cases of explosive trauma. Hence, for barotraumata the statistical correlation must by necessity be less clear.

The Schwartze-Eysell experiments of 1873 had not addressed themselves to differences in damping [435].

(2) Ruptures of Shrapnell's membrane are rare because it displacements are generally of small magnitude [488]. Although the membrane is rather flaccid, the limited volume of the attic and the narrow communication with the ME proper apparently provide sufficient damping.

4. Lesions of the Ossicular Chain

The occurrence of traumatically induced lesions of the ossicular chain has been recognized for quite some time. The first description of an incudostapedial discontinuity was given by *Toynbee* in 1866 [cited after 19]. *Barnick* [20], in 1897, reported another such case. From a literature survey, *Passow* [339] collected 13 cases of fractures of the mallar handle. They had been produced either by direct, transmeatal injuries or by blunt skull traumata. *Passow* assumed that the malleus, being the most lateral ossicle, would be more easily injured than the other two. He furthermore cited 2 cases of incus luxation produced via the EEC. He was also the first to report on an iatrogenic lesion of that kind incurred during the course of mastoid surgery. *Schwartze* [382] as well as *Passow* [339] recognized the fact that a foreign body entering the middle ear via the EEC could push the stapes footplate into the vestibule, and that such a dislocation would cause vestibular signs and symptoms as well as hearing loss.

Sakai [369] and *Lange* [262] conducted postmortem examinations on patients who had died after a skull trauma. In a total of 9 autopsies, *Sakai* found 7 ossicular-chain lesions, most of them combinations of incudomallar disruptions and stapes fractures. *Lange* saw 3 incudomallar luxations in a series of 20 cases. Despite this rather clear evidence, the notion of *Ulrich* [443] prevailed, at least for some time, i.e. that skull traumata would not produce ME injuries in an indirect manner. In only 2 out of 22 postmortem examinations, *Ulrich* found that the 'ossicles had been dislodged from their normal position' but, in his opinion, there was no discontinuity. *Ulrich*'s debatable notion was not even abandoned after *Voss* [450] had published his monograph that summarized his own findings made during the course of surgery of the otobasis. *Voss* documented a number of cases in which he found ossicular-chain defects of traumatic origin. Finally, *Kelemen* [230] showed again that ossicular lesions might well be produced in this manner: he clearly demonstrated incudomallar disruptions that had occurred after blunt skull traumata.

It took 13 more years until the tympanoplastic principles were applied to the reconstruction of ossicular chains damaged by trauma, principles that had originally been developed for the restoration of the sound-conducting system after defects of *infectious* origin. Even as late as 1956, *Proctor* et al. [352], in their survey, *The Ear in Head Trauma*, failed to mention that posttraumatic hearing losses might be due to ossicular lesions. *Plester* [347] and *Thorburn* [432a], independently in 1957, published their first reports about the surgical correction of posttraumatic ossicular lesions. *Plester* described 3 cases in which he had successfully repositioned the incus that had been luxated earlier during the courses of simple mastoidectomies. *Thorburn* carried out type III tympanoplasties to correct the fixation of the mallar head and the luxation of the incudostapedial joint; both had been produced by blunt skull traumata.

A few years later, a large number of papers had appeared on the above topic, enabling *Escher* [99] and *Kley* [248] to present their surveys on a large variety of lesions of the ossicular chain and to list the methods of reconstruction recommended by various authors.

4.1. Causes of Ossicular Lesions

Posttraumatic ossicular-chain lesions are caused in general by the same kinds of trauma that produce TM lesions. However, the frequencies of occurrence are not equal in the 2 cases. *Schwartze* [382] and *Passow* [339] mentioned already that transmeatal insults, caused for instance by foreign bodies, misguided attempts of extraction of a foreign body or myringotomies, if perforating the TM in its posterosuperior quadrant, may also injure the incudostapedial joint or the stapes. *Armstrong* [13] reported on 15 such cases and *Silverstein* et al. [397] on 9 more. Both authors pointed out the potential danger inherent in lesions in this part of the TM. In most cases, however, it is the *lower* quadrants of the TM that are being damaged (cf. chapter 3.4.3).

During the course of a simple mastoidectomy, the incus might be inadvertently luxated, thereby interrupting its joints with the two adjacent bones [138, 339, 347, 395, 464]. Such accidents occurred especially in the premicrosurgical era.

Extreme displacements of the TM may lead to an overextension of the incudostapedial joint, and thus to its disruption, as *Helms* [187] was able to observe in experiments on guinea pigs. (However, the guinea pig is prone to such injuries, since it lacks the incudomallar joint which, when mobile, is capable of absorbing some of the incident, low-frequency energy [496].) Clinical findings of this kind were reported by *Lesoine* [265] and *Teodorescu* et al. [428]. For example, while the EEC was being irrigated, ossicles were disrupted, although the TM remained intact. These, as well as other similar defects seen after barotrauma, although occurring quite rarely, might have been caused by the mechanism just described. Lesions produced by explosions occurred more frequently on account of the much stronger incident force [81]. Most of them were found in combination with TM ruptures [262, 296].

Most authors consider the blunt skull trauma the most frequent cause of ossicular-chain injuries [65, 99, 163, 204, 248]. Contrary to *Ulrich*'s [443] notion, already mentioned, they reasoned that the impact ought to exert a remote effect on the ME system. This in turn could produce lesions of the ossicular chain, TM ruptures or a combination of both of them. Frequently, but by no means invariably, lesions of the ME mechanism were found after TB fractures [262, 369]. However, such fractures were also found without any involvement of the ME [262, 361, 438, 443] and, conversely, ME lesions were seen without fractures of the skull base [61, 163, 224].

Reports vary considerably about the incidence of ME involvement in patients with blunt skull trauma. *Willis* [464], in a series of 50 blunt skull injuries, found no such case. *Cremin* [65] gave an incidence of 1% for all his cases with blunt skull trauma, *Guerrier* et al. [163] 15%. (These included several cases of transient deafness.) *Glaninger* [139] found 8 cases with ossicular defects in a total of 235 TB fractures (3.4%), *Tos* [439] 29 in a total of 222 (13%) and *Rohrt* [361] 9 in a total of 120 (7.5%). *Rohrt* gave the incidence of TB fractures as 6–8.4% for his series, *Lundin* et al. [274] as 7.5% in a total of 899 skull fractures. The relative frequency of laterobasal fractures among all skull fractures is said to be higher after traffic accidents (21%) than after other forms of skull traumata (7.5%) [274]. Furthermore, modern methods of resuscitation and intensive care have improved the chances of patient survival after skull trauma. Some authors therefore believe that, in recent years, the frequency of ossicular-chain defects is rising together with the increase in motorization [224].

The foregoing discussion points to a causal relation between blunt skull trauma and injuries to the ossicular chain, a relation that can no longer be denied. Nevertheless, the nature of the underlying mechanism is still under discussion. *Hough and Stuart* [204] listed several events that may produce ossicular-chain lesions, either individually or in combination: (1) tetanic contractions of the ME muscles; (2) vibratory impulses caused by strong impacts; (3) ossicular inertia that becomes effective during periods of positive or negative accelerations of the entire head, and (4) fractures of ME structures that are brought about when the ME walls are split during the course of longitudinal TB fractures and the fragments move apart.

To avoid confusion, it should be mentioned that, *in its normal mode of vibrations*, the ossicular chain displays a very low moment of inertia [481]. However, accelerations *of the entire head* could be a different matter, as will be discussed in chapter 4.6 later on.

Kley [248] considered the above point No. 4 of *Hough and Stuart* [204] especially important. He felt that some ossicular disruptions might represent direct extensions of fracture lines entering the tympanic annulus. He also pointed out that fractures of the tympanic roof might cause the ossicles to be pushed into the direction of the hypotympanum.

A discussion of the underlying mechanism(s) will be postponed until after presentation of the Tübingen findings (chapter 4.6).

4.2. Locations of Ossicular Injuries

Traumatic injuries of the ossicular chain may manifest themselves in three different forms or their combinations [81, 248]: (1) luxations; (2) fractures, and (3) fixations.

Fixation is the end result of adhesions, calcification of the ossicular ligaments or of direct contact of fractured or luxated bones with the ME walls [61].

Which form of lesion will result in a given case is determined by the kind and direction of the incident force, the reaction of the ME and the resistance of the various parts of the ossicular chain against injury. Table XXVII (after [138]) lists the average resistance of the various sections of the chain against their being torn or fractured. This table indicates that the incudostapedial joint is the weakest link of the chain, followed rather closely by the incudomallar joint. The resistances of the annular ligament and of the stapedial crura are nearly identical, being clearly higher than those of the joints.

Dürrer et al. [85, 86], by means of photoelastometry, determined in an ME model the courses of stress lines resulting from forces acting upon the frame of the tympanic cavity and its contained structures from a generally lateral direction. The strongest stresses were found to be generated in the incudomallar joint and in the incudostapedial one, followed in decreasing

Table XXVII. Limiting force at which various parts of the ossicular chain are torn or fractured (after [138])

	Limiting force, g
Annular ligament	177
Stapedial crura	166
Incudostapedial joint	52
Long incudal crus	674
Incudomallar joint	67
Incudomallar and incudostapedial Joints combined	119

order by the long process of the malleus, the stapes footplate and the crura. (Experiments of that kind permit one only to state, where stresses will be greatest, not necessarily, where luxations and/or fractures will occur. That will also depend on the detailed internal structure of the bones, ligaments or joint capsules, something that cannot be readily duplicated in a model experiment.)

The malleus is held in place by its intimate connection with the TM [Graham, personal communication, 1982] and by the tendon of the tensor-tympani muscle, the stapes by the annular ligament and the stapedial tendon. The incus, however, is only weakly held in place by the ligaments in the incudal fossa and at the tympanic roof and by the joints with its two neighboring ossicles [248, 395]. It follows therefore that most disruptions ought to involve the incus. According to the statistical survey of Hammond [173], the incus was involved in 73% of all ossicular-chain lesions, the stapes in 29% and the malleus in only 16%. (Since there were some multiple lesions, the total exceeded 100%.) Luxation of the incudostapedial joint is the injury most frequently seen. It was found in 10 out of 16 cases of ossicular-chain defects [65]. Others saw nothing but this lesion (5 cases [157]; 4 cases [242]; 1 case [448]). Hough and Stuart [204] gave its incidence as 82.3% in a total of 31 cases. The luxation seen next in frequency is that of the incudomallar joint or that of the incus at both of its joints (8 cases out of a total of 17 [1]; 6 out of 13 [80]; 2 cases [195]; 1 case [29]; 1 case [389]). In these lesions, the incus was occasionally dislocated and thrown into an osseous cleft created by a TB fracture or even under the skin of the external canal [137, 162, 464].

Traumatically induced luxations of the stapes into the vestibule are rare. They can only occur when the annular ligament is torn — and that ligament is rather strong. Such luxations are caused by forces that act directly across the ME in a generally medial direction [51, 158, 292, 343, 464]. The stapes may be completely torn out of the oval window, but that form of injury has only rarely been encountered [21, 326, 428].

The malleus was occasionally found torn off the backside of the TM, its ligaments being simultaneously disrupted; the pull of the tensor tympani had presumably dislocated it in an anteromedial direction [99, 194].

Fractures were found less frequently than luxations, but all three ossicles may be involved. Fractures of the stapes footplate have been described. They were produced either directly [472] or by blunt skull trauma; in the latter case, there were usually concomitant fractures of one or both crura [8, 66, 194, 368, 409]. Isolated fractures of the crura close to their insertion at the footplate were seen rather frequently. *Marquet* (in a discussion of [444]) believed that such fractures occur only in the presence of an otosclerotic stapes fixation; in that case, the mechanical impact would strike a rigid structure rather than a yielding one. In otosclerosis, furthermore, the crura are supposed to be often quite thin and thus mechanically more vulnerable than normal. *Marquet* [444] reported on 11 cases of stapedial fractures of his own; in all of them otosclerosis was demonstrated histologically; 6 of the patients firmly denied the occurrence of an earlier head trauma.

Similar cases have been described [33, 65, 296, 322]. *Plath* [346] and *Jackson* [213] both reported on incus luxations, or fractures, respectively, in patients with otosclerotic stapes fixation. On the other hand, *Does and Bottema* [80] saw crural fractures in 4 patients with clearly mobile stapedes. Similar findings were reported by others (2 cases [8]; 11 cases [93]; 2 cases [321]; 3 cases [444]). Two of these authors [80, 93] mentioned that the lesion in question was seen mainly in younger patients: 3 children of a total number of 4 patients [80] and 7 of 11 [93].

Teodorescu et al. [427] thought that such a lesion might be brought about by a severe downward tilt of the stapes, while the incus is being pushed in the direction of the hypotympanum in the manner described by *Guerrier* et al. [160, 163]. Thereby, the crura could be shorn off or the annular ligament torn, especially in its anterior portion, where the fibers are not only longer [470], but also thinner than those of the posterior portion (300 vs 500 μm) [49]. The same mechanism might also be responsible for jerking the stapes completely out of the oval window, leaving it standing on the promontory [8]. Theoretically at least, it could also produce a fracture of the stapedial neck, an apparently rare lesion, since it has only been described twice [65, 463].

Incus fractures were seldom seen. When found, they always involved the long crus, close to the lenticular process (3 cases [65]; 1 case [120]; 2 cases [138]; 1 case [224]; 1 case [428]). Apparently, such lesions may also interfere with the blood supply of this region, eventually leading to a necrosis of the long incudal crus [32].

Hamberger and Wersäll [172] as well as *Lindeman* [268], mentioned that the long crus possesses a rather poor blood supply. In addition to some vessels that cross over from the stapes head via the mucoperiosteal cover [*Bast*, cited after 435], the long crus receives only one or a few more thin vessels from the incudal body. Any interruption of these vessels therefore introduces the danger of an ischemic necrosis of the long crus.

Malleus fractures are also rare, contrary to the opinion of *Passow* [339], who, as is recalled, considered the malleus the most vulnerable of all ossicles. There are only a few reports on fractures of the mallar handle between the umbo and the short process [56, 99, 222, 248, 424] and on fractures of its neck [163, 202, 287, 397, 453]. In guinea pigs, mallar fractures were rather frequently found after explosions [492]. The reason for the latter finding is the missing protection by the incudomallar joint that was already described (cf. chapter 4.0).

Finally, the ossicular chain, even when left structurally intact, may be impaired in its mobility by pressure exerted on it from the outside, for example by cerebral prolapses [163, 249] or by an arachnoidal cyst [249]. More frequently, such impairment is caused by scars due to adhesions, following mucous membrane lesions, or due to the fibrous replacement of a hemotympanum [139, 249, 409]. Adhesions may ossify, when fragments of the tympanal wall come in contact with the ossicles [61, 464]; but ligaments may also ossify after having been overstretched, especially those around the mallar head [65, 80, 195, 432] and in the incudal fossa [80, 287, 389]. Posttraumatic ossification of the annular ligament presents a special diagnostic problem. The fixation might have indeed occurred subsequent to a trauma or the footplate might have already been fixated prior to it, thus facilitating the injury of the ossicular chain (cf. above). In 2 cases, in which the crura were fractured and the footplate fixated, there was little doubt that both changes were induced by the same trauma, since the surgeon found the footplate in a slanted position within the window [427]. In other cases, a traumatic origin was made at least probable by the patient's history [43, 58, 60, 66, 139].

4.3. Signs, Symptoms and Diagnosis of Ossicular Lesions

The leading sign of ossicular lesions is a conductive hearing loss. Its magnitude may vary between 20 and 50 dB [92, 248], depending on whether ossicles are healed in a structurally good position or in a poor one — although in the latter case the function may accidentally be quite satisfactory [80] — or whether the chain is completely discontinuous behind an intact TM.

The tentative diagnosis of a posttraumatic ossicular lesion requires first that an adequate trauma had actually taken place: a transtympanic injury, a blast trauma, or a blunt head trauma, or that a simple mastoidectomy had been performed earlier. To make the diagnosis probable in the case of a blunt head trauma, *Hough and Stuart* [204] demanded that there should have been loss of conciousness, bleeding from the ear and hearing loss. Although this triad of signs and symptoms is found rather frequently, its occurrence is not absolutely mandatory. Quite a large number of cases with lesions of the ossicular chain have been described, in which the skull trauma had been relatively mild; no loss of consciousness had occurred, there was no evidence for a fracture of the TB, neither was there a TM rupture and thus bleeding from the EEC had not occurred [61, 163, 224].

The otoscopic findings during the early stages following a *transtympanal* injury are quite characteristic: there is a fresh TM perforation, significantly in the *posterosuperior* quadrant [13]. Covering it fails to improve hearing [224]. Early examination of skull-trauma patients with concomitant ME injuries, on the other hand, does not always provide one with a set of unequivocal clues. The finding that the TM is intact, or is torn in extension of a fracture line through the tympanic annulus, does not reveal anything about the state of the ossicles. There is usually a hemotympanum, which by itself could account for the hearing loss present. Only when the hearing loss persists for 4–6 weeks or even longer, even though the tympanic cavity has again been properly aerated and the TM has regained its normal appearance [377], the existence of an ossicular lesion should be suspected [248].

In the rare case of a fractured mallar handle, otoscopic findings are quite unambiguous, since its abnormal mobility is easily demonstrated with the aid of a Siegle otoscope [222]; likewise in those cases in which a dislocated incus can be discerned through the TM [99, 389] or when it is found lying under the skin of the external canal [137]. There may of course be some indirect evidence pointing to a preceding trauma, such as a step in the osseous wall of the EEC, scars in the TM or a surgical retroauricular scar [1, 81, 395].

X-Ray pictures are of limited value. Not every longitudinal TB fracture can be visualized on Schüller projections [66, 135, 137, 248, 317, 361, 438]. Moreover, it is only in a small percentage of such fractures that the ossicular chain is injured [438]. On the other hand, ossicular defects may exist in the presence of intact TB [61, 163, 224, 368, 447].

Tomography is occasionally helpful. It aids in demonstrating a luxated incudomallar joint or a missing long incudal crus. Tomographic reports were found to agree with clinical findings in 11 of a total of 21 cases [9], in 29 of 50 cases [92], in 22 of 34 cases [214] and in 80% of 205 cases [447]. (In all of them the tympanic cavity had been found normal and well aerated.) In some cases, however, tomography does not reveal a luxated incudostapedial joint, the most frequent of all lesions [56], or a stapedial fracture [9, 93, 134, 135, 321, 395, 429]. The audiometric examination remains therefore the most important diagnostic measure. A pure conductive hearing loss or a mixed loss (types I or II of *Escher* [99]), together with an appropriate history and a normal or near-normal appearance of the TM should let one suspect an ossicular lesion, especially when the hearing loss is confined to the side of the original injury and when it has remained stable for some time [9, 395]. Bilateral ossicular defects following blunt skull trauma have been reported [34, 369], but they appear to be rare.

Demonstration of an abnormally mobile TM by means of impedance testing may indicate an ossicular discontinuity. Nevertheless, this test has little, if any, value in cases of subluxation or fixation of some parts of the chain [66, 173]. Failure to demonstrate a stapedial reflex by impedance audiometry may indicate a fixation or a discontinuity lateral to the incudostapedial joint [56, 81]. However, when the crura are fractured but the remaining chain is mobile, the stapedial-reflex test may yield a false-positive result [8, 56, 93]. When the incudomallar joint is disrupted, there may be a larger-than-normal impedance change, which is due to the elicitation of the tensor-tympani reflex [92].

If the mallar head is fixated, the bone-conduction audiogram decreases toward 2,000 Hz but, as a rule, it stays flat, failing to return toward the higher frequencies, as it does in the case of the classical Carhart's notch. This pattern was observed in patients [484] as well as in experimental animals [495].

The cochlear symptoms are not characteristic. Tinnitus may occasionally be evoked by a pure ME lesion [56, 61, 339, 464] as well as by a cochlear lesion. A pure sensorineural hearing loss (type III of *Escher* [99] is usually a sign of a coexisting cochlear trauma [365]. Fluctuating hearing losses and concomitant vertigo may point to the existence of a perilymphatic fistula in the region of either window. (Since they represent special cases, perilymphatic fistulae, including luxations of the stapes footplate, will be discussed separately in chapter 7.)

There is a consensus of opinion [65, 81, 92, 163, 173, 199, 248, 287, 321, 359] to the effect that the diagnostic measures described merely serve to raise the suspicion that an ossicular lesion may exist, but that they do not provide positive proof. Only an exploratory tympanotomy will yield that information. If and when the suspicion is corroborated, surgery may immediately be extended for the correction of the defect found.

4.4. Management

4.4.1. Spontaneous Healing

A luxated joint may heal spontaneously, provided the joint surfaces reappose themselves in a satisfactory manner. This type of healing has been demonstrated in animal experiments [403]. It was also observed clinically, i.e. an incus previously luxated had successfully repositioned itself [56, 99, 347, 359].

It was repeatedly observed that a narrow gap persisting between the two surfaces of the incudostapedial joint was bridged by strands of scar tissue, thus providing at least some continuity and facilitating the transmission of sound, albeit in an attenuated form [65, 80]. Following spontaneous healing or surgical repair, the joint(s) may be filled with scar tissue to varying extents, but this must not necessarily impair sound conduction to a measurable degree [403]. This demonstrates the well-known fact that, while the chain is vibrating in response to audiofrequencies, at least the incudomallar joint is completely immobile [481] — but then, there is the danger of ossicular fractures when displacements become excessive (cf. above).

Spontaneous healing that leads to a persistent structural defect and yet permits a fair transmission from the TM to the cochlea is apparently rare. *Does and Bottema* [80] described such an occurrence (their case 5). The incus was luxated in both joints; but its body had accidentally established contact with the head of the stapes, and the long crus was firmly attached to the tympanal surface of the TM. The incus thus acted as a columella. There was a conductive hearing loss of less than 20 dB. The entire situation was detected by chance during the course of a surgical FN decompression. Another type of spontaneous repair that has been repeatedly described is that the TM becomes firmly attached to the head of the stapes in the manner of a type III tympanoplasty [e.g. 65]. The spontaneous healing of a luxated stapes footplate will be described in some detail in chapter 7.

It is difficult to estimate how many ossicular luxations may heal spontaneously. During the early stages, the hearing loss present might be attributable to the hemotympanum that almost invariably exists. When the latter has been completely resorbed, after 4–6 weeks [377], the joint may have conceivably restored itself sufficiently so that there is no longer a detectable hearing loss. When the ME happens to be explored for some other reasons (e.g. FN paralysis, otogenic meningitis) soon after the trauma, one might occasionally find a freshly torn joint capsule without dislocation of the ossicles. Hence, these are only accidentally observed.

Opinions are still divided as to the question whether or not ossicular fractures may heal spontaneously. Little is known about mallar fractures. Von Troeltsch [cited after155] described his finding of a fractured mallar neck that had spontaneously healed. *Passow* [339] thought that mallar fractures could heal spontaneously, but he did not submit any relevant data. *Voss* [450], quite accidentally, found a healed fracture of the mallar handle several years after the original trauma. *Jungmayr* [222], on the othe hand, saw a pseudarthrosis 5 years after such a fracture. Other authors [56, 99, 248, 424] also described fractures of the mallar handle, but did not address themselves to the above questions.

Spontaneous healing of a fractured long incudal crus has never been described, only its posttraumatic necrosis [32], as was already mentioned in chapter 4.2.

Stapedial fractures were the subject of many studies in several animal species: cats [403]; cats and monkeys [26], and rabbits [7]. They were also studied in stapedial tissue cultures from guinea pig and man [50]. According to these experiments, fractured crura as well as fractured footplates appear to have a good tendency to heal. However, *Altmann and Basek* [7] did not convince themselves that these experimental results would also apply to the human case. They based their opinion on a report by *Wolff and Bellucci* [470] who, at the occasion of an autopsy, found a well-healed fracture of the footplate; nevertheless, a concomitant crural fracture did not show any callus formation. *Burton and Lawrence* [50] did not find evidence of ongoing repair in their human tissue culture preparations either, but they expressed the belief that the human stapes should not be different in this respect from the guinea pig stapes, in which they had found callus. And then again, *van den Eekhaut* [444] was of the opinion that none of the human ossicles are capable of forming any callus since, in contrast to other bones, their growth is already completed during the 22nd fetal week. Moreover, *Lindeman* [268] pointed out that the stapedial crura possess a minimal blood supply in the region just above the footplate, the place of predilection of their fracture.

Waltner et al. [455] had the opportunity to examine two human temporal bones, 26 or 46 years respectively after stapes footplate fractures. Both of them had been incurred during ME surgery. These authors found the fragments in the enchondral layer held together by scar tissue, but genuine callus only in the periosteal layer. They failed to make any statements regarding the state of the crura. *Martin* et al. [291] perforated footplates surgically in some cases of Menière's disease. (There was *no* otosclerotic fixation.) In 6 of their cases, the window was closed over by newly formed bone. Hence, such closures do not only occur when there is otosclerosis in the oval window (OW) region, as had been frequently claimed in the early days of fenestration surgery. *Van den Eekhaut* [444] was unable to find any evidence of callus formation in, or the healing of, fractured crura, neither in 3 cases of his own nor in any others reported in the literature. Even in papers published since then, no such cases have been described [34, 93, 326, 368, 472].

Summarizing at this point, one may state that spontaneous healing of fractured stapedial crura and footplates was demonstrated in animal studies. In humans, callus formation was found only within the periosteal layer of the footplate, not in the enchondral layer [455]. Furthermore, ankylosis has been described after footplate fractures and luxations. There is no clear-cut evidence for the spontaneous healing of a fractured malleus, of an incus or of the stapes superstructure.

It was never reported that the mobility of an ossicular chain, once it had been impaired by scar tissue or by newly formed bone, was spontaneously restored — nor should one expect such an occurrence.

For all the reasons given, the treatment of choice of most posttraumatic ossicular luxations and of all fractures and fixations is surgical intervention.

4.4.2. Surgical Management

The aim of ME surgery in cases of ossicular-chain defects is the restoration of a functional conductive system and thus the improvement of hearing. Therefore, the indication for surgery is essentially determined by the audiometric findings. On the one hand, the conductive component of the hearing loss present must be large enough so as to make a postsurgical improvement probable. From this standpoint, the minimal presurgical loss has been said to be approximately 20dB [65, 139]. On the other hand, there must be a sufficient cochlear reserve so that one may expect a useful gain in hearing. Extreme sensorineural hearing loss or even complete deafness, as found after transverse fractures, but occasionally also after labyrinthine concussions with or without longitudinal fractures, are contraindications for the surgical exploration of the ME [99]. Perilymphatic fistulae are the exception from this rule, as will be discussed later in chapter 7. Only a few authors believe that posttraumatic tinnitus is an indication for ossicular-chain surgery [339, 464].

There is a consensus of opinion about the *timing* of surgery. It should not be performed too early. Neither from the audiological standpoint [377], nor from the roentgenological one [447], can a diagnosis of ossicular-chain discontinuity be made, not even a tentative one, until the aeration of the tympanic cavity has been restored and its mucoperiosteal lining has completely healed, i.e. for a period of about 4–6 weeks. There are some authors who believe that the inner ear might be sensitized by trauma and might react to subsequent surgery more strongly than usual. *Glaninger* [139] and *Kley* [248] therefore expressed the opinion that one should wait for 3–6 months before performing an exploratory tympanotomy. Even longer waiting periods are not known to constitute a disadvantage: defective ossicular chains were successfully repaired in a number of cases many years after the original trauma. There is only one exception from this rule: one should not postpone a surgical repair if at the occasion of an earlier intervention, necessitated for other reasons (e.g. posttraumatic FN paralysis; CSF leakage from the ear; meningitis of otogenic origin), an ossicular-chain defect is found accidentally or when a perilymphatic fistula is detected that was produced by the luxation or fracture of the stapes footplate.

A large number of different methods has been recommended for the surgical reconstruction of a damaged ossicular chain. Some authors with extensive series of cases point out that the surgeon should always make his decision on an individual basis, since each case represents a unique situation [19, 56, 173, 204].

Simple repositioning of the incus is all that is usually needed to correct its luxation in either one of its two joints [56, 80, 347, 397]. Scarification of the joint surfaces leads to a stable union with the adjacent bone(s) [56, 120]. If the incus is fixated by connective-tissue adhesions or by osseous fusions, repositioning will not be possible until these adhesions or fusions are lysed. Pulling a C-shaped wire loop through the obturator foramen and crimping it over the long incudal crus [199, 259, 260] or putting a polyethylene sleeve around both of them will prevent the lenticular process from recoiling [99]. *Dietzel* [77] uses a piece of vein for that purpose. If a gap exists between the lenticular process and the stapedial head some surgeons advocate to bridge it by interposing a piece of connective tissue [80], small pieces of bone [9, 195,

202, 464], cartilage [66, 321], polyethylene tubing [19, 65, 139, 173] or by means of tissue glue [56].

The simplest corrective procedure for a completely luxated incus that is disconnected from both of the adjacent bones is to lower the TM onto the stapes head in the manner of a type III tympanoplasty [22, 432, 463]. Based on theoretical considerations about the mass loading of the oval window, *Portmann* [351] and *Elbrond* [92], independently, recommended to interpose the incus between stapes head and mallar handle, after cutting it down in size. *Andersen* et al. [9] and *Hough* [202], however, employed the incus in its unaltered form. Other materials that are being used for the same purpose include the mallar head [80, 248], cartilage transplants [224, 406, 445] or the proplast prosthesis developed by *Shea* [173].

A luxated, but mobile stapes footplate should be carefully repositioned [61, 292]. However, if it is broken or the crura are fractured, stapedectomy is the method of choice. The procedure is basically the same as that used in otosclerosis surgery [66, 173, 343, 368].

The surgical management of fractures of the mallar *handle* has not been described. *Silverstein* et al. [397] performed a type II tympanoplasty in a patient with a fractured mallar *neck*.

Attempts to use a small piece of bone for splinting a fractured long crus of the incus, e.g. fastening the two together by means of polyethylene rings [*Marquet*, cited by 56], or employing a piece of polyethelene tubing sleeved over the bones [428], remained unsuccessful. In such cases, *Chalat* [56] recommended to carry out an incudostapediopexy, simply wiring the two pieces of bone together, if it were at all structurally possible, or to extract the incus and to reposition it between mallar handle and stapes head. *Kley* [248] preferred a direct malleostapediopexy; to this end, he rotated the malleus backwards. *Hociota* et al. [195] employed essentially the same procedure wiring the two bones together.

A number of surgeons, when finding the stapedial crura fractured but the footplate intact, do not like to extract it for fear of creating an additional trauma in the inner ear [173]. *Yanagisawa* et al. [472], in 1 such case, successfully repositioned the fractured crura, supporting them with gelfoam. *Does and Bottema* [80], in 2 cases, employed connective tissue for the same purpose. *Elbrond and Aastrup* [93] were able to preserve the footplate in 11 cases of crural fractures; in 3 of them, they maintained their position by interposing bone chips, in others, they put a piece of polyethylene tubing between incus and footplate or interposed the incus itself. *S. Muñoz Borge and Marco* [321] placed cartilage between incus and footplate. Others [43, 248] crimped a wire around the long crus of the incus and positioned its other end on the mobile footplate. Still others [21, 65, 359] performed a stapedectomy, followed by an incudovestibulopexy, or malleovestibulopexy with the aid of a wire and vein graft. For cases with extensive destruction of the ossicular chain, involving the incus as well as the stapes superstructure, *Kley* [248] employed a type IV tympanoplasty, i.e. he put the TM directly in contact with the footplate. Other authors, in attempting to maintain the lumen of the tympanic cavity, constructed a columella, positioning either the long crus of the incus onto the footplate [56, 202] or interposed a piece of polyethylene tubing [80]. *Chalat* [56] as well as *Hough and Stuart* [204] gave some thought to the possibility of transplanting a homologous TM and ossicular chain in such cases.

Surgical methods suitable for the repair of ossicular fixations have not been described. As was pointed out by some authors, one ought to sever adhesive scars [139, 194, 409]. However, it was only *Kley* [248] who stressed the fact that one should always try to preserve the mucous membrane in such a procedure or to cover defects by small grafts. If the footplate is fixated, stapedectomy is recommended, to be executed in the manner of otosclerosis surgery [61, 213, 222, 428]. Fixations of the mallar head should be lysed and osseous epitympanal bridges be severed [195] or they should be bypassed by resection of the mallar head and the incudal body. Thereafter, the ossicular chain should be rebuilt according to the principles just outlined — if a direct myringostapediopexy would not be preferred [65, 99].

A survey of the results achieved is difficult to present. In most papers, only single cases are described, the mode of injury and the surgical method employed varying widely from paper to paper. Moreover, the postsurgical audiometric results were not presented in a uniform manner. Only a few larger statistics are available. In some of them [92, for example], no distinction was made between ossicular defects of traumatic origin and those of infectious origin. In spite of these shortcomings, an attempt will be made in the following to present the various modes of reconstruction according to their functional aspect. The results achieved will be listed in terms of the average gain at the audiometric speech frequencies and of the remaining impairment, both rounded off to the nearest 5 dB. If a given author presented a number of similar cases, his best and worst results will be cited and the averages be given in parentheses.

For their 31 cases, *Hough and Stuart* [204] described the absence or persistence of a conductive loss, less than 10 dB in magnitude, but only in terms of percentages (table XXVIII).

Table XXVIII. Conductive losses remaining after various surgical procedures in percent (after [204])

Procedure	Conductive loss <10 dB	No loss remaining
Ossicular repositioning (n = 5)	80	60
Malleostapediopexy (incus on stapes head) (n = 6)	100	0
Malleoplatinopexy (incus interpositioned) (n = 5)	80	60
Incudolabyrinthopexy (wire) (n = 2)	50	0
Malleolabyrinthopexy (n = 3)	100	100
Tympanoplasty type III (n = 1)	0	0
Other methods (n = 9)		

According to tables XXIX to XXXVII, almost identical audiometric results were achieved by the various procedures for repositioning the incus, by malleostapediopexies with elongation of the stapes head and by myringostapediopexies; the remaining conductive impairment was about 11–13 dB. Putting a bridge between the lenticular process and the stapedial head gave slightly lesser results; the remaining conductive impairment was about 15 dB. Connecting incus and footplate (sometimes executed by repositioning a fractured stapedial crus) gave excellent results: the average remaining deficit was only 10.5 dB. Incudovestibulopexy resulted in an average postoperative gain of 29 dB, the remaining loss being about 7 dB. However, this procedure produced at least one completely dead ear [80]. Results of connecting the malleus directly with the footplate or the vestibule respectively were somewhat less satisfactory; the remaining loss was 11 or 12 dB, respectively. Nevertheless, these results were not worse than those obtained by the various methods that preserve the stapes superstructure or those that are employed after luxation of the incudostapedial joint.

Table XXIX. Results of repositioning the incus (median values in parentheses)

Author	Number of cases	Audiometric gain, dB	Remaining conductive loss, dB	Remarks
Cremin [65]	4	15–30 (20)	0–15 (10)	polyethylene fixation
Does and Bottema [80]	4	0–20 (15)	10–45 (20)	
Elbrond [92]	1	10	10	
Escher [99]	5	5–45 (25)	0–15 (5)	polyethylene sleeve (one)
Flisberg and Floberg [120]	1	40	20	
Holler and Greenberg [199]	1	40	0	wire fixation
Kuschke [260]	1	45	0	wire fixation
Spector et al. [409]	5	–5–25 (10)	10–30 (20)	
Total	22	–5–45 (20)	0–45 (12)	

Table XXX. Results after repositioning the stapes (median values in parentheses)

Author	Number of cases	Audiometric gain, dB	Remaining conductive loss, dB
Chvojka and Mrovec [61]	1	30	20
Teodorescu et al. [428]	1	20	25
Schwetz [389]	2	10–20	20–30
Silverstein et al. [397]	1	?	20
Total	5	10–30 (20)	20–30 (23)

Table XXXI. Results after incudostapediopexy and elevation of the stapedial head (median values in parentheses)

Author	Number of cases	Audiometric gain, dB	Remaining conductive loss, dB	Remarks
Andersen et al. [9]	1	25	?	bone
S. Muñoz Borge and Marco [321]	1	35	10	cartilage
Cummings [66]	1	30	0	cartilage
Does and Bottema [80]	1	20	15	jelly
Elbrond [92]	8	10–20 (15)	5–45 (20)	bone, polyethylene
Hociota et al. [195]	1	50	0	bone
Vilar-Puig et al. [448]	1	20	20	polyethylene
Willis [464]	1	20	5	bone
Total	15	10–50 (21)	0–45 (15)	

Table XXXII. Results after incudoplatinopexy (median values in parentheses)

Author	Number of cases	Audiometric gain, dB	Remaining conductive loss, dB	Remarks
Armstrong [13]	1	40	10	stapedial crura repositioned
Does and Bottema [80]	2	10–30	15	stapedial crura repositioned
Elbrond [92]	8	10–55 (25)	0–25 (5)	ossic. reposition-ing, polyethylene
Spector et. al. [409]	6	0–30 (10)	5–30 (10)	wire and polyethylene
Yanagisawa et al. [472]	1	40	0	stapedial crura repositioned
Total	18	0–40 (21)	0–30 (10.5)	

Table XXXIII. Results after incudolabyrinthopexy in the absence of otosclerosis; (median values in parentheses)

Author	Number of cases	Audiometric gain, dB	Remaining conductive loss, dB	Remarks
Bartlett [21]	1	30	0	steel wire
Bicknell [33]	1	60	5	steel wire
Bouchayer and Mereaud [43]	1	20	5	Shea piston
Campbell [51]	1	25	20	steel wire
Charachon et al. [58]	1	40	10	Teflon piston
Chvojka and Mrovec [61]	1	40	0	steel wire
Cremin [65]	6	20–40 (30)	0–20 (10)	steel wire and Teflon
Cummings [66]	5	20–30 (25)	0–10 (5)	steel wire
Does and Bottema [80]	1	dead ear	—	polyethylene
Van den Eeckhaut [444]	2	25–35	0	teflon piston
Hociota et al. [195]	1	35	0	polyethylene
Jackson [213]	1	30	10	Shea piston
Nakano and Ishikawa [326]	1	30	20	cartilage
Pellerin and Poncet [343]	1	?	15	polyethylene
Sadé [368]	2	35–40	0	steel wire
Silverstein et al. [397]	1	20	10	steel wire
Spector et al. [409]	1	25	5	
Teodorescu et al. [428]	2	20–25	10–15	polyethylene, stapes position inverted
Vilar-Puig et al. [448]	1	20	10	
Total	31	20–60 (29)	0–20 (7)	

Table XXXIV. Results of tympanoplasty, types II and III (median values in parentheses)

Author	Number of cases	Audiometric gain, dB	Remaining conductive loss, dB	Remarks
Andersen et al. [9]	1	35	?	type III
Bauer [22]	1	40	5	type III
Cremin [65]	1	25	0	type III
Does and Bottema [80]	1	35	5	type III
Elbrond [92]	2	10–45	10–15	type III
Escher [99]	5	10–25 (20)	10–15 (15)	type III
Flisberg and Floberg [120]	2	15–25	25	type III
Glaninger [139]	1	20	35	type II
Kirikae et al. [242]	4	25–35 (30)	10–20 (15)	type II (three) type III (one)
Silverstein et al. [397]	1	25	10	type II
Spector et al. [409]	3	10–25 (20)	5–15 (10)	type III
Williams [463]	1	30	10	type III
Schwetz [389]	2	20–35	5–15	malleus transposition
Total	25	10–45 (26)	0–35 (13)	

The worst results from the functional standpoint were, by a wide margin, those obtained after repositioning the stapes in the OW; the remaining auditory impairment was usually in excess of 20 dB.

Elbrond [92] and Spector et al. [409], independently, examined the question if the postsurgical audiometric results would alter with time. Both authors observed that, even when the reconstructed ossicular chain functioned well initially, years later the conductive impairment often increased again.

Summarizing the present chapter, we might state that the probability of keeping the postsurgical audiometric deficit smaller than 20 dB after the repair of a variety of ossicular defects is rather good, regardless of the method employed — the only exception being the repositioning of a luxated stapes. Glaninger [139] and Cremin [65] stated, correctly in our opinion, that an exploratory tympanotomy is justified, whenever a traumatically induced ossicular lesion is suspected and the conductive impairment is in excess of 20 dB.

Table XXXV. Results of tympanoplasty, type III with elevation of stapes head (median values in parentheses)

Author	Number of cases	Audiometric gain, dB	Remaining conductive loss, dB	Remarks
Andersen et al. [8]	1	20	?	incus
S. Munoz Borge and Marco [321]	1	35	15	incus
Does and Bottema [80]	2	15–35	15–20	mallar head, polyethylene
Elbrond [92]	84	0–60 (25)	0–50 (10)	incus, bone, polyethylene
Glaninger [139]	4	20–30 (25)	15–25 (20)	polyethylene
Hociota et al. [195]	2	25–30	5–15	wire and polyethylene
Junien-Lavillauroy et al. [224]	1	20	5	cartilage
Spector et al. [409]	2	15–20	0–15	incus
Willis [464]	2	10–20	15–40	wire
Total	99	0–60 (26)	0–50 (11)	

Table XXXVI. Results of malleoplatinopexy (median values in parentheses)

Author	Number of cases	Audiometric gain, dB	Remaining conductive loss, dB	Remarks
Armstrong [13]	1	25	0	incus
Cummings [66]	1	25	25	incus
Does and Bottema [80]	1	40	10	Teflon
Elbrond [92]	41	0–55 (25)	0–45 (10)	malleus, incus, bone, polyethylene
Spector et al. [409]	4	0–45 (25)	10–25 (20)	wire
Total	48	0–55 (27)	0–45 (12)	

Table XXXVII. Results of malleolabyrinthopexy

Author	Number of cases	Audiometric gain, dB	Remaining conductive loss, dB	Remarks
Cremin [65]	2	25–30	0–5	wire-Teflon
Glaninger [139]	1	10	30	steel wire
Messervy [296]	1	25	10	steel wire
Total	4	10–30 (22.5)	0–30 (11)	

4.5. Our Clinical Results and Postmortem Findings

4.5.1. Causes – Age and Sex Distribution

The present series included 144 patients with posttraumatic ossicular lesions. In 134 cases, the diagnosis was confirmed during the surgical exploration of the ME. In 2 additional patients, a fracture of the malleus handle was seen otoscopically, but surgical intervention was not warranted. Sound transmission was normal in 1 of them; in the other, there was a small deficit, less than 20 dB. In 8 other patients, the history and the clinical findings strongly suggested the existence of an ossicular defect, but the recommended surgery was refused. Therefore, confirmation of the diagnosis was not feasible, nor was it possible to pinpoint the exact site of the suspected lesion.

Blunt skull trauma was by far the most frequent cause of ossicular disruption: 108 cases (75%). With a much lesser frequency, it was the result of an iatrogenic artifact: 19 cases (13%). Next in line were transtympanal traumata (direct mechanical or blast injuries): 15 cases (10%). In 2 cases (2%), a preceding trauma was denied. Included in the group of transtympanal traumata were 10 injuries produced by explosions and 2 more caused by slaps on the ear, making a total of 12 blast injuries. There were 3 mechanically caused TM perforations that involved the ossicular chain; they were respectively produced by a hair pin, a knitting needle and a cotton tip.

16 of the 19 iatrogenic artifacts had been produced in the course of simple mastoidectomies performed during childhood. In 1 more case, the incus had been luxated during a stapedectomy. In another case, the incudostapedial joint

had been interrupted during the extraction of a foreign body from the EEC and, in the last one, the stapedial crura were broken during cleansing of an ear, in which a wire malleostapediopexy had been carried out earlier.

To separate the ossicular defects caused by blunt skull traumata from those caused by laterobasal skull fractures appeared to be a rather futile task, according to what was already stated. Basically, both types of injury are produced by the same kinds of insult and occur frequently in combination.

Table XXXVIII therefore analyzes 190 patients by cause of injury and by age and sex. In these patients, either an ossicular-chain defect had occurred in the absence of a homolateral skull fracture (27 cases: 14%) or a TB fracture was present, without damage to the ossicular chain (82 cases: 43%); finally, both kinds of injury had taken place in combination (81 cases: 43%). The relative incidence of ossicular-chain lesions in the present material, i.e. in about 50% of all cases of TB fractures, is probably too high for the general case. Only those patients were seen clinically who displayed overt otological symptoms; those with uncomplicated laterobasal skull fractures were never seen and were therefore not included in the present survey.

No bilateral ossicular-chain injuries were observed. In 3 cases of longitudinal TB fractures, however, a luxation of the incudostapedial joint (1 case) or of both incudal joints (2 cases) existed, which happened to be in the *contralateral* ear.

Among all cases of blunt skull trauma, traffic accidents (111 cases) were much more frequent than injuries sustained while falling or being hit (76 cases). Gunshot injuries hardly played a role – quite understandably in peacetime. Only in 3 such patients, all of them injured during WW II, was there an ossicular defect.

Inspection of table XXXVIII indicates that three quarters of all patients injured in traffic accidents, by falling or by being hit, were male. For traffic accidents, the incidence was highest between the 11th and 30th years of life and for the two other kinds between the 21st and 50th years. Many of these were probably the result of industrial accidents, since the age of most patients fell into the range of the average work age. Female patients were injured by falling mainly during childhood or at higher ages. At either end of the age scale, the frequencies of occurrence for both sexes approached each other.

10 of the transtympanal traumata were caused by explosions. All patients were males between the ages of 5 and 36 (average age 20 years). Injuries caused by slaps on the ear were found in 1 woman, aged 34, and in 1 man, aged 25. The mechanical injuries had occurred in 2 women, aged 23 and 39, respectively, and in a boy of 7.

Table XXXVIII. Age and sex distribution of laterobasal head injuries (82 temporal-bone fractures, 27 ossicular defects, 81 combined injuries). Absolute figures with percentages given in parentheses

	Age, years							
	0–10	11–20	21–30	31–40	41–50	51–60	61–70	71–80
A. After falling or being hit (n = 76)	12 (16)	7 (9)	10 (13)	20 (26.5)	10 (13)	7 (9)	9 (12)	1 (1.5)
Males (n = 59; 77%)	7 (12)	5 (8.5)	9 (15)	19 (32)	8 (13.5)	5 (8.5)	5 (8.5)	1 (2)
Females (n = 17; 23%)	5 (29)	2 (12)	1 (6)	1 (6)	2 (12)	2 (12)	4 (23)	–
B. Traffic Accidents (n = 111)	12 (11)	36 (32)	33 (30)	10 (9)	11 (10)	7 (6)	1 (1)	1 (1)
Males (n = 79; 71%)	8 (10)	24 (30)	25 (32)	7 (9)	8 (10)	5 (6)	1 (1.5)	1 (1.5)
Females (n = 32; 29%)	4 (13)	12 (38)	8 (25)	3 (9)	3 (9)	2 (6)	–	–
C. Gunshot injuries (n = 3; all male)	–	1	1	1	–	–	–	–
Total (n = 190)	24 (13)	44 (23)	44 (23)	31 (16.5)	21 (11)	14 (7.5)	10 (5)	2 (1)
Males (n = 141; 74%)	15 (11)	30 (21)	35 (25)	27 (19)	16 (11.5)	10 (7)	6 (4)	2 (1.5)
Females (n = 49; 26%)	9 (18.5)	14 (29)	9 (18.5)	4 (8)	5 (10)	4 (8)	4 (8)	–

Most of the simple mastoidectomies responsible for ossicular lesions had been performed in children between the ages of 2 months and 16 years (medium age 6 years). Only 1 patient was already 27 years old. The sex distribution was equal (8 to 8).

The incudomallar luxation that had resulted from a foreign-body extraction had occurred in a girl of 4. The cleansing of the previously operated ear had been carried out in a 14-year-old.

It may be recalled from chapter 4.2. that some authors [80, 93] saw isolated fractures of the stapedial crura mainly in children. In the present series, there were 9 such fractures. None of the patients was younger than 10 years; 2 were between 10 and 20 years and 2 others between 20 and 30. This finding appears to contradict those of the authors just mentioned. However, when one correlates all ossicular-chain defects and TB fractures (except those caused by gunshots) with the patient's age at the *time of the injury*, one gains the impression that disruptions of the ossicular chain might occur more frequently during childhood and that isolated temporal-bone fractures were more frequent during higher ages (table XXXIX).

Table XXXIX. Ossicular defects and temporal-bone fractures: the effect of chronological age. Absolute figures with percentages given in parentheses

	Age, years			
	0–10	11–20	21–30	> 30
Ossicular defects without temporal-bone fractures (n = 27)	4 (15)	10 (37)	7 (26)	6 (22)
Ossicular defects in the presence of temporal-bone fractures (n = 79)	13 (17)	19 (24)	19 (24)	28 (35)
Temporal-bone fractures without ossicular defects (n = 81)	7 (9)	14 (17)	17 (21)	43 (53)

4.5.2. Symptomatology

The history of the patient and his audiometric findings give the strongest indications for the existence of an ossicular-chain defect. As already mentioned, a preceding trauma of adequate magnitude was missing in the history of only 2 of our 144 patients. In 2 other patients, there was no conductive impairment. In 1 of these, a fractured malleus handle was found on otoscopic inspection. In the other, there was a luxation of the incudostapedial joint that had repaired itself on its own. (Because of its interesting features, this latter case will be discussed in greater detail later in chapter 4.5.6.)

In addition to the patient's history, the findings made under the otomicroscope and the results of the audiometric examination constituted the most important diagnostic criteria. Roentgenological examinations were limited to the standard projections of *Schüller* and of *Stenvers*. Occasionally, lateral-skull X-rays were available; they had been taken for the verification of fracture lines and will be discussed in that connection. Tomographic examination was not performed because of its limited diagnostic value with respect to the lesions under discussion.

Ossicular defects caused by blunt head trauma were the exception from the rule: in only some of these cases did the otoscopic examination provide useful information. In 51 of the 81 cases of longitudinal TB fractures with concomitant ossicular injuries, i.e. in 63%, the TM appeared entirely normal. TM perforations were found in only 25 ears (31%). The remaining 5 TM (6%) showed scars. In 46 cases (57%), a step in the osseous wall of the external canal pointed to the existence of a longitudinal fracture. In 20 of the 27 patients with ossicular lesions but without signs of longitudinal fractures (which were not even demonstrated during surgery), i.e. in 74%, the TM appeared entirely normal. In 4 cases there were scars in the TM (15%) and in the 2 remaining cases a perforation (7.5%). An epitympal cholesteatoma was discovered in 1 ear; according to the surgical findings, however, it had probably nothing to do with the preceding skull trauma.

As inspection of table XL indicates, TM scars were only found in association with traumata that had occurred some times in the past. Although direct evidence was lacking, they could conceivably represent remnants of traumatic ruptures that had spontaneously healed. Nevertheless, since in many cases the appearance of the TM was described as being completely normal, even a few days or weeks after the trauma, one may assume that ossicular injuries often occur without damage to the TM. This assumption was corroborated by the fact that the ratio between perforated TM and intact ones (last line of table

XL) remained constant over time, indicating that most TM had never been ruptured.

It goes without saying that in all cases of transtympanal injuries the TM must have been initially perforated. Otoscopic inspection revealed existing perforations in 7 TM (47%), scars in 7 others (47%). 1 intact TM was found (6%) that, following a blast injury, was no longer connected to the mallar handle. In 2 cases of ossicular lesions (1 incus luxation and 1 fractured stapedial crus, both of unknown causes) the TM was intact and appeared normal.

No TM injuries had apparently been inflicted in those cases in which the ossicular chain had been damaged during the course of ME surgery. Neverthe-

Table XL. Tympanic membrane findings in patients with ossicular-chain lesions associated with head trauma.

	Time interval after trauma				
	0–3 weeks	4–6 weeks	7 weeks to 3 months	4–12 months	> 1 year
A. With longitudinal temporal bone fracture (n = 81)					
TM perforation (n = 25)	8	3	1	4	9
Scars in TM (n = 5)	–	–	–	—	5
TM intact (n = 51)	15	5	2	7	22
Ratio of perforated/intact TM	4/7	4/6	3/7	4/6	3/7
B. Without temporal-bone fractures (n = 27)					
TM perforation (n = 2)	–	–	–	–	2
Scars in TM (n = 4)	–	–	–	1	3
TM intact (n = 20)	2	1	2	2	13

Epitympanal cholesteatoma (n = 1)

less, one must expect that some perforations ought to have existed due to the original infection. At the time of the examination, only 1 central perforation was found, 40 years after a simple mastoidectomy, and 1 scarred TM after an earlier surgical removal of a foreign body.

For 13 patients, no presurgical pure-tone audiograms were available. 11 of them had undergone emergency surgery on account of a skull-brain trauma. Their condition before surgery had not permitted an audiological examination. The 2 others were children, who were also submitted to emergency surgery on the suspicion that the stapes might have been depressed into the vestibule by a force acting via the tympanic cavity. Table XLI presents the pure-tone audiometric findings in all patients, separately for conductive and sensorineural components. The second column, labeled 'other traumata', includes transtympanal injuries, iatrogenic ones and those of unknown causes. The sensorineural function was considered normal when either the impairments did not exceed the limits given by patient's age and/or when the hearing levels were symmetrical on both sides. A loss beyond these limits was considered evidence of a sensorineural impairment. It was of course not possible to exclude old noise-induced impairments with certainty. The division: (a) no sensorineural hearing loss; (b) moderate to severe sensorineural hearing loss, and (c) complete deafness, corresponds approximately to *Escher*'s [99] categories I–III. (However, Escher's type III also includes severe sensorineural impairments.) On complete-

Table XLI. Audiometric (pure-tone) findings in patients with ossicular chain lesions

Pure-tone audiogram	Blunt skull traumata (n = 108)	Other traumata (n = 36)
1 Data not available	11	2
2a Conductive loss 0–20 dB	15	2
2b Conductive loss 20–30 dB	32	9
2c Conductive loss > 30 dB	43	23
3a No sensorineural loss	36	8
3b Sensorineural loss moderate to severe	44	20
3c Profound sensorineural loss	7	–
4 Carhart's notch type II	10	6

ly deaf ears, surgery was carried out, if at all, only for unrelated causes and the ossicular-chain lesions listed were found accidentally during such interventions. One is forced to conclude that, most likely, ossicular-chain injuries occur more frequently than table XLI indicates in ears that, at the same time, are rendered completely deaf.

The last category of impairment in table XLI is labeled 'Carhart notch type II', to distinguish it from that usually seen in otosclerosis. This type II notch was found in 16 patients (11%) with ossicular discontinuities (cf. table XLI).

Since the Carhart notch type I is eliminated after stapedectomy, or is at least made smaller, the postsurgical fate of the type II notch was also examined (table XLII). 2 of the patients in question did not show up for the control examination. In 2 others (1 incus luxation and 1 fracture of the stapedial neck), the notch had completely disappeared postsurgically; in 6 more patients it had become smaller, without vanishing completely. This clinical observation confirms earlier findings in experimental animals [495], but is at variance with the opinions of several other authors [81, 92, 395, 444].

Table XLII. Postsurgical sensorineural function in patients with Carhart's notch, type II

Lost to follow-up (n = 2)	Normal (n = 2)	Improved (n = 6)	Unchanged (n = 6)
		3 patients with incudostap. luxation	5 patients with incudostap. luxation
1 patient with incus luxation	1 patient with incus luxation 1 patient with stap. neck fracture		
		1 patient with fractured stapedial crura	
1 patient with incudostap. luxation and stap. luxation		1 patient with incudostap. luxation and fixation of mallar head	1 patient with malleus fracture, incudostap. luxation and fractured stap. crura
		1 patient with incus luxation and fractured malleus	

The point must be stressed that Carhart's notch of either type *never* indicates the presence of a sensorineural lesion, but merely that the EEC and ME components of bone conduction, for a variety of different reasons, fail to reach the cochlea [495].

Impedance audiometry was carried out in 26 patients. In 20 of them, the results were corroborated during subsequent surgery. That is to say, in 19 cases of ossicular-chain discontinuity the stapedial reflex could not be elicited. In 5 of the remaining patients, in whom surgery also revealed an ossicular discontinuity, an impedance change was registered, which was wrongly considered a positive stapedial reflex. In reality, probably, these either represented tensor-tympani reflexes or artifacts. There was a positive reflex in 1 patient with a stapes luxation, but the reflex was negative in another patient with fracture of the stapes crura, where the stapedius muscle was in contact with the intact part of the ossicular chain. This obviously was also a false-negative result.

Tympanometry was carried out in only 7 patients. In 4 of them, the results agreed with the surgical findings: 1 was a TM of normal mobility, but with a subluxated incudostapedial joint; another was a TM braced by a fixated mallar handle and the 2 last ones were extremely mobile, in 1 case due to a fracture of the mallar handle and in the other due to a luxation of the incus. In 3 cases, the impressions gained during surgery did not seem to agree with the results of the preceding measurements: 2 of the TM were described as being stiff and 1 as appearing normal, although in all 3 cases a luxation of the incudostapedial joint was present. (But then again, mere clinical impressions are not always reliable.)

4.5.3. Locations of Ossicular Lesions: Clinical Patients

Surgery was carried out in 100 cases of ossicular-chain lesions caused by blunt skull trauma and in 36 more cases of various other causes. The intervention permitted the exact determination of the site of the defect. The analysis of these sites will start with the cases caused by blunt head injury. Added to this series might be the 2 cases of fractured malleus handles. Although they were not treated surgically, the diagnosis was clearly established by otoscopy. 21 of these 102 cases had multiple chain injuries. The 81 singular lesions are presented in table XLIII and the 21 multiple lesions in table XLIV.

According to table XLIII, the majority of the singular chain lesions (62 of 81) involved the joints of the incus with its 2 neighbors. Although these lesions were more frequently found in conjunction with TB fractures, they occurred also in their absence. It appears therefore that TB fractures do not necessarily predispose to ossicular-chain injuries of a distinct type.

Table XLIII. Sites of 81 singular ossicular-chain disruptions after head trauma

Type of lesion	Total number of cases	In the presence of TB fractures	In the absence of TB fractures
Incudomallar luxation	10	7	3
Incudostapedial luxation	28	24	4
Incus totally luxated	24	21	3
Stapes luxation	2	2	0
Fractured malleus handle	3	1	2
Fractured incus	2	2	0
Fractured stapes	9	6	3
Ossicular fixation	3	3	0
Total	81	66	15

Only those cases in which the footplate had been actually moved out of its normal position were counted as stapes luxations. Mere perilymphatic fistulae in the OW area will be discussed separately in chapter 7.

In 1 case of an incudal fracture, the distal end of the long crus and the lenticular process had remained connected to the head of the stapes, while the body of the incus was missing. In a second case, the situation was reversed, i.e. the long crus was completely absent, but the body had remained in situ. In both cases, evidently, the long crus of the incus had been fractured off the body. 8 of the stapes fractures involved the crura, 1 of them the footplate.

In 3 cases, the mallar head was fixated, in 1 of them also the incus. All of them were osseous fixations in the region of fracture lines in the tegmen tympani.

In contrast to the singular lesions, most of the multiple lesions (table XLIV) had occurred in conjunction with longitudinal TB fractures, i.e. with homolateral fractures (18 cases), with a contralateral fracture (1 case) and with a contralateral gunshot injury (1 case). It was in only 1 patient (luxation of both incus and stapes and osseus fixation of the incus), that no TB fracture could be demonstrated.

Table XLIV. Sites of multiple ossicular-chain interruptions in 20 patients

	Malleus fracture	Incudomal-lar luxation	Incudo-stapedial luxation	Incus luxation	Stapedial fracture	Stapedial luxation	Ossicular fixation
1	+	+					
2	+		+				
3	+		+				
4	+			+			
5	+			+			+
6		+					+
7		+					+
8			+		+		
9			+		+		
10			+		+		+
11			+		+	+	
12			+				+
13			+				+
14				+	+		
15				+	+		
16				+	+	+	
17				+		+	
18				+		+	
19				+		+	+
20				+			+
Total 5		3	8	9	7	5	8

Not listed in table XLIV is a case with a combined fracture of the long incudal crus and of both stapedial crura as well as a separation of the mallar handle from the TM (case 21). Three of the mallar fractures involved the manubrium, 2 its neck. The stapedial crura were broken in 6 cases, the neck in 1 and the footplate in still another. In 4 of the 8 cases of *osseous fixation,* the mallar head was fused to the attic walls. In 2 others, the luxated body of the incus was firmly attached to the lateral attic wall. In 1 more case, the stapes was hardly mobile; there were connective-tissue adhesions and the incudosta-pedial joint had been luxated. In the eighth case, a piece of bone had been blown out of the posterior wall of the external canal, pressing onto the incus and restricting its mobility; but there was no osseous fusion.

Injuries of the ossicular chain caused by direct transtympanal insults presented a similarly diverse picture (table XLV; the 2 lesions of unknown causes are included in here).

All mallar fractures listed in table XLV involved the handle, those of the stapes the crura. In 2 of the osseous fixations, the malleus head was found fixated in the attic; in 1 case, the stapes footplate was fixated.

There were 19 cases of ossicular disruption of iatrogenic origin. 16 of them had been produced during the course of simple mastoidectomies. 1 patient refused surgery. In the remaining 15, the following lesions were found:

	Cases
Luxation of the incudostapedial joint	5
With simultaneous stapedial luxation	1
Complete luxation of the incus	4
With simultaneous fixation of the mallar head	2
Luxation of the incus (missing at the time of surgery)	2
Fracture of the stapedial neck	1
Total	15

The remaining 3 iatrogenic lesions included the following: a fracture of the stapedial crura, brought about during the cleansing of the ear canal in an ear in which a malleostapediopexy had been performed at an earlier time (this case has already been mentioned); 1 incus luxation incurred during stapedectomy, and 1 luxation of the stapes and of the incudostapedial joint; both had occurred during the removal of a foreign body from the ear canal.

The various ossicular-chain lesions and their relative frequencies were thus found to be quite similar for a variety of different kinds of injury. Hence, there is no trauma that predisposes to a lesion in a certain part of the ossicular chain.

Table XLVI gives the location and relative incidence of all 172 ossicular defects seen in 138 patients. (In this table, each lesion that was part of a multiple injury is entered as a separate entity.) It is seen that more than two thirds of all ossicular-chain defects were luxations, mainly of the incus (61%).

Ossicular fractures represented less than one fourth of all lesions. They involved mainly the stapes, less frequently the malleus and only occasionally the long crus of the incus.

Table XLV. 17 cases of ossicular defects caused by transtympanal traumata

	Mallar fracture	Incudo-mallar luxation	Incudo-stapedial luxation	Incudal luxation	Stapedial fracture	Stapedial luxation	Ossicular fixation	State of TM	Cause
1	+		+		+			scarred	explosion
2	+			+				perforated	explosion
3	+						+	scarred, separated from mallar handle	explosion
4			+					scarred	knitting needle
5			+					scarred	explosion
6			+					perforated	explosion
7			+		+			perforated	hair pin
8				+				scarred	explosion
9				+				perforated	not known
10				+				intact	slap on the ear
11					+			perforated	slap on the ear
12					+			scarred	not known
13					+			intact	Q-tip
14						+		perforated	explosion
15							+	perforated	explosion
16							+	scarred	explosion
17								intact, separated from mallar handle	explosion
Total	3	0	5	4	5	1	3		

Table XLVI. Incidence of all types of ossicular lesions (n = 172). Absolute figures with percentages given in parentheses

Malleus handle separated from TM	3 (2)		
Incudomallar luxation	13 (7.5)		
Incudostapedial luxation	48 (28)	105 (61)	118 (69)
Incus totally luxated	44 (25.5)		
Stapedial luxation	10 (6)		
Fractured malleus handle	9 (5)	11 (6)	
Fractured mallar neck	2 (1)		
Fractured long incudal crus	3 (2)		38 (22)
Fractured stapedial neck	2 (1)	24 (14)	
Fractured stapedial crura	20 (12)		
Fractured footplate	2 (1)		
Fixation of mallar head	11 (6)		16 (9)
Fixation of incus	3 (2)		
Fixation of stapes	2 (1)		

Posttraumatic fixations were relatively rare and concerned mainly the mallar head. There is hardly any doubt that fixations develop gradually. It would be quite conceivable therefore that the incidence of fixations might increase with the time elapsed between the original trauma and the date of surgery. A survey of the present cases based on this notion showed that the earliest intervention for a malleus fixation was carried out 2 months after the time of the trauma, the latest after 44 years. The average was 16 years. Included in this group was the patient mentioned earlier, in whom the mobility of the incus was severely impaired by a piece of bone impinging on it; however, even after 21 years no real adhesion had formed. In the remaining cases, in which no fixation or osseous fusion had taken place, the average interval between trauma and surgery was 8 years with a rather wide variation in time. 21 operations were performed during the first month, 24 more before the end of the first year. On the other extreme, 14 operations were carried out after an interval of more than 20 years, the longest being 70 years. One may assume therefore that the waiting period plays only a minor role in the generation of fixations. More important might be other factors, such as a firm contact between the ossicles and the osseous walls of the ME cavity, especially when there were lesions of the mucoperiosteal lining caused by the original trauma.

4.5.4. Locations of Ossicular Lesions: Postmortem Specimens

The examination of 89 temporal bones, removed immediately after death that was directly caused by a severe skull trauma, revealed 18 longitudinal and 2 transversal TB fractures, 2 atypical in direction and 1 in an ear with an old radical mastoid cavity. (This latter case was not further evaluated because of the absence of the ME structures.) Ossicular-chain lesions were found in 4 of the longitudinal fractures and in 1 transversal fracture. 2 such defects were detected in cases *without* TB fractures. Both, however, had suffered severe skull traumata: In 1 of them, there was a homolateral fracture in the cranial vault and a second fracture in the region of the posterior fossa; in the other case, there was a TB fracture on the contralateral side. This last case was the only one of the entire series in which there were *bilateral* postraumatic ossicular-chain lesions.

Hence, there were 2 specimens with ossicular lesions, but without TB fractures, 5 with such lesions and simultaneous TB fractures and 17 with TB fractures, but with intact ossicular chains. In terms of relative frequency, the ratios were 8:21:71%. In the *clinical* series (chapter 4.5.1), the percentages had been 14:43:43%, or 27:81:82 in absolute numbers.

The relative incidence of pure TB fractures was thus considerably higher in the postmortem material than in the clinical series. This possibility had already been alluded to in the discussion of the clinical results (chapter 4.5.1). It stands to reason that the routine assessment of uncomplicated TB fractures in clinical patients must by necessity be less reliable than that in postmortem specimens.

In contrast to the foregoing, the ratio of ossicular lesions without TB fractures to their combined occurrence was approximately equal in both series. It was 28.5:71.5% for the postmortem material and 25:75% for the clinical series.

In the postmortem material, there were 5 ossicular-chain defects among the 22 TB fractures found, a percentage of 23%. As such, the incidence was considerably higher than the 13% reported by *Tos* [438] for his *clinical* series. *Rohrt* [361] found not more than 9 ossicular-chain interruptions in his series of 120 TB fractures (7.5%). For TB fractures as percentages of *all* blunt skull traumata, he gave incidences of 6% or 8.4%. *Lundin* et al. [274] gave a figure of 7.5%. If one takes the latter value, which lies between *Rohrt*'s two percentages, one may extrapolate the present postmortem findings in the following manner: one ought to expect ossicular-chain interruptions in 23% of all TB fractures but also in some cases of blunt skull trauma without skull fractures. In the present series, the incidence of TB fractures was 5.75% of all specimens examined and that of ossicular-chain defects 25% of all TB fractures, indicating that there might be an ossicular-chain lesion in about 2% of all blunt skull traumata. This figure is somewhat higher than the 1% reported earlier by *Cremin* [65].

The ossicular lesions found in the postmortem material were distributed as follows:

Associated with longitudinal fractures — fracture of the mallar handle and incus luxation; fracture of the stapes neck; luxation of the incudostapedial joint (tegmen tympani torn off, together with malleus and incus); luxation of the incus in the presence of an otosclerotic footplate fixation.

Associated with a lateral transversal fracture — fracture of the stapes footplate and of the anterior crus.

In the *absence* of TB fractures — luxation of the incus and fracture of the anterior stapedial crus; luxation of the incudostapedial joint.

Table XLVII presents a summary of all ossicular lesions associated with blunt skull traumata that were found in the postmortem material. Since all injuries were quite fresh, no fixations had yet taken place.

The autopsy material included the only case of the entire series, i.e. patients *and* postmortem specimens combined, in which an ossicular-chain lesion (incus luxation) existed in the presence of an otosclerotic stapes fixation, a combination that was relatively often described by other authors (cf. chapter 4.2). It must be mentioned in this connection, however, that the incidence of fractures was about 50% higher in the postmortem material than in the clinical series.

Table XLVII. Postmortem material (n = 10): ossiculr lesions associated with blunt skull trauma

Incudostapedial luxation	2 ⎱	5 (50%)
Total incudal luxation	3 ⎰	
Fractured mallar handle	1 (10%)	
Fractured stapedial neck	1 ⎱	
Fractured stapedial crura	2 ⎰	4 (40%)
Fractured footplate	1 ⎰	

The ossicle that was most frequently luxated was the incus (50%), but it was the stapes that was most frequently fractured (40%). On account of the small numbers, however, one cannot expect a better agreement between the series of postmortem specimens and the clinical series.

4.5.5. Clinical-Surgical Management

Spontaneous healing of ossicular fractures was never observed. However, in 1 case, a temporarily separated incudostapedial joint had spontaneously reunited itself. This was accidentally detected during surgery for a perilymphatic fistula. Presurgically, there had been a small conductive impairment of a mere 10 dB. One may safely assume that luxations repair themselves rather frequently without being recognized clinically, since ears of this kind are usually not submitted to surgery, unless there are some other reasons, as the fistula of the present case. Counted in the same category should be: (a) the 2 cases of fractured mallar handles, which did not require surgical corrections because the auditory function was good (conductive impairments of 0 and 20 dB, respectively); (b) 2 other cases, in which the long crus of the incus had attached itself to the TM as in a type II tympanoplasty. In 1 of the latter patients, surgery had not been required either, since the average conductive impairment amounted to only 7 dB. In the other case, with a conductive impairment of 18 dB, a luxated incudostapedial joint was detected at the time of surgery.

In 136 patients, attempts were made to surgically reconstruct the ossicular chain. TM perforations, if they existed, were closed by scarifying their margins and by putting autologous fascia onto their tympanic surfaces (cf. chapter 3.3.3). Because of the wide variations in the type of lesions observed, surgical procedures were selected that were most suitable for each given case, i.e. procedures, which required the least alterations of any parts of the conductive system that were still present and appeared structurally and functionally sound. Table XLVIII presents a survey of the procedures selected and the relative frequency of their use. The incus was only repositioned if it could be easily brought into its normal position and remained there without special fixation.

In 2 dead ears, the OW niche was covered with fascia and the stapes footplate placed onto this graft. In a third case with a still functioning ear, the stapes that had been depressed into the vestibule was lifted up. The torn annular ligament was covered with small pieces of connective tissue.

The methods most frequently used for ME rconstruction after incus

Table XLVIII. Surgical procedures employed for reconstruction of the ossicular chain (n = 136)

Incus repositioning	5 }	8
Stapes repositioning	3 }	
Malleostapediopexy (autologous incus)	46	
Malleostapediopexy (homologous incus)	30	
Malleostapediopexy (mallar head)	2	
Malleostapediopexy (proplast prosthesis)	2 }	87
Malleostapediopexy (ceramic prosthesis)	2	
Malleostapediopexy (wire)	4	
Myringostapediopexy (tympanoplasty, type III)	1	
Incudoplatinopexy (wire)	5	
Incudoplatinopexy (Teflon piston)	1	
Malleoplatinopexy (autologous incus)	2	
Malleoplatinopexy (homologous incus)	5 }	16
Malleoplatinopexy (ceramic prosthesis)	1	
Malleoplatinopexy (wire)	2	
Incudovestibulopexy (wire)	2	
Incudovestibulopexy (Teflon piston)	1 }	7
Malleovestibulopexy (wire)	4	
Mobilization of mallar head	2 }	3
Mobilization of stapes	1 }	
No reconstructive procedure	15	

luxation were various forms of malleostapediopexy. The patient's own incus was usually employed. Only when it was too severely damaged a homologous bone preserved in Cialit was used. The incus was either positioned with its short crus parallel to the mallar handle and a small groove was cut into its other end for fitting it onto the stapes head; or two grooves were cut, one of which was placed on the mallar handle and the other onto the stapedial head. Other materials that were occasionally employed for the same purpose included the mallar head or prostheses made of proplast, ceramic of aluminum oxide, or of wire. In only 1 case was the TM directly placed on the stapes head.

When the stapes superstructure was missing but the footplate was mobile, an incudovestibulopexy was carried out, either with the aid of a Schuknecht wire prosthesis or with that of a Guilford wire-Teflon piston. The piston was sometimes positioned onto the footplate after the latter had been carefully shattered. When both incus and stapes were found damaged the gap between the mallar handle and the footplate was bridged by an incus

— either the patient's own or a homologous one — the long crus being placed onto the footplate. In 1 such case, a ceramic prosthesis, in 2 others, wire prostheses were used to the same end.

Footplates, when mobile and intact, were preserved if at all possible (in 16 cases). It was only when the footplate had been luxated, fractured or was immobilized, that it was removed (in 7 cases). In such cases again, either the prosthesis of Schuknecht or that of Guilford served as replacement as in a routine stapedectomy.

Fixated mallar heads were remobilized successfully in 3 cases, thus preserving ossicular continuity. In 15 cases, reconstructive measures were not carried out at all, because the ear in question was dead, or not immediately, because additional surgery was planned for a later date, for example for the treatment of a posttraumatic cholesteatoma.

4.5.6. Surgical Results

Serious postsurgical complications were not encountered. *Structural* failures included the following: (a) recurrence of TM perforations in 3 cases. 2 of them healed subsequently after surgical revisions; (b) one postsurgical cholesteatoma, and a second recurring one; both of them were successfully removed at a later time; (c) excessive scar formation in the middle ear (1 case) after its walls had been severely shattered and the middle-ear space was largely oblitered by scar tissue.

The following represent *functional* failures: (a) deterioration (in 4 cases) of ME conduction that had initially been good. Surgical revisions uncovered renewed discontinuities as the original replacements had slid out of position; (b) deterioration of ME conduction in 2 cases by 8 or 4 dB, respectively. No surgical revisions were undertaken. In 2 other cases, the posttraumatic conductive impairment persisted after surgery without a change; (c) a transient sensorineural impairment following malleovestibulopexy by means of a homologous incus (1 case). The auditory function recovered on Rheo-macrodex-novocaine infusions and sympathetic-ganglion blockage.

Audiometrically, the surgical results may either be assessed in terms of the auditory gain achieved or in terms of the remaining (conductive) impairment. The latter is often the better indicator, since the auditory gain is largely determined by the magnitude of the presurgical, conductive hearing loss. The auditory gain was determined by comparing the pre- and postsurgical averages for the five frequencies of 0.25, 1, 2, 4, and 8 kHz. The remaining, conductive hearing loss was assessed in accordance with the rules given in chapter 3.4.9 in connection with table XXII. In some of the present patients, postsurgical audiograms were not available so that neither the auditory gains nor the remaining hearing losses could be determined. The results obtained in the remaining 81 patients are presented in table XLIX. The following symbols are employed: MS = malleostapediopexy; IP = incudoplatinopexy; MP = malleoplatinopexy; IV = incudovestibulopexy, and MV = malleovestibulopexy.

In addition to the cases listed in table XLIX, 1 stapes (audiometric gain 27 dB, remaining conductive impairment 0 dB) and 1 malleus head (audiometric gain 12 dB, remaining conductive impairment 14 dB) were mobilized.

Results, optimal with respect to the audiometric gains as well as to the remaining conductive impairments, were achieved by repositioning a disarticulated incus, by malleostapediopexy (ceramic or wire prosthesis), incudoplatinopexy (wire prosthesis), malleoplatinopexy (ceramic prosthesis) and by incudovestibulopexy (Teflon prosthesis). However, some of the favorable results were only obtained in single cases and may thus be wholly accidental. The results achieved with the aid of autologous and/or homologous incudes appeared to be equally good from the statistical standpoint. Although ceramic and wire prostheses seemed to give better results, their superiority could not be confirmed statistically because of the small number of cases (t-test > 5%). Their relative superiority might again be wholly accidental.

To provide a better summary, table L presents the same surgical results once more, but in an abbreviated form, i.e. under neglect of some technical details. A perusal of the table indicates that, in terms of the remaining impairment, results appeared to be best after the reconstruction of the ossicular chain either by repositioning or by mobilization. Next in line came the stapedial replacement (incudoplatinopexy or incudovestibulopexy). Substitution of the incus (malleostapediopexy) and of both, incus and stapes (malleoplatinopexy or malleovestibulopexy), fared relatively poorest, although the average remaining impairment in the last two instances was still better than 20 dB. (Again, the numbers of cases under most of the entries are rather small, making the information somewhat uncertain from the statistical standpoint.)

Tables XLIX and L show that in cases of suspected ossicular discontinuities ME surgery is indicated if the presurgical conductive impairment is larger than 20 dB. Under that condition, the probability of achieving a useful auditory gain is good, regardless of which method might turn out to be best suited for the case at hand.

Table XLIX. Audiometric results after surgical correction of ossicular defects

Procedure and number of patients	Audiometric gain, dB				Remaining conductive loss, dB			
	min	max	av.	SD	min	max	av.	SD
Incus repositioned (n = 5)	6	31	16	± 10	0	15	6	± 8
MS (autologous incus) (n = 32)	-4	39	13	± 10	0	38	18	± 9
MS (homologous incus) (n=20)	-8	53	19	± 15	0	45	19	± 10
MS (mallar head) (n = 1)	–	–	3	–	–	–	15	–
MS (PORP) (n = 1)	–	–	16	–	–	–	17	–
MS (ceramic) (n = 2)	25	30	27	± 4	0	15	7	± 10
MS (wire) (n = 2)	30	40	35	± 7	10	14	12	± 3
IP (Wire) (n = 3)	8	23	17	± 8	5	17	9	± 7
IP (Teflon piston) (n = 1)	–	–	14	–	–	–	15	–
MP (autologous incus) (n = 2)	2	4	3	± 1	11	29	20	± 13
MP (homologous incus) (n = 4)	0	32	16	± 15	0	47	19	± 20
MP (ceramic) (n = 1)	–	–	38	–	–	–	0	–
MP (wire) (n = 1)	–	–	13	–	–	–	22	–
IV (wire) (n = 2)	13	18	15	± 4	21	22	21	± 1
IV (Teflon piston) (n = 1)	–	–	41	–	–	–	9	–
MV (wire) (n = 3)	30	30	30	–	0	37	16	± 19

Table L. Summary of audiometric results after surgical correction of ossicular defects

Surgical procedure and number of patients	Audiometric gain, dB				Remaining conductive loss, dB			
	min	max	av.	SD	min	max	av.	SD
Ossicular repositioning (n = 6)	6	31	16	± 10	0	15	6	± 8
Ossicular mobilization (n = 2)	12	27	19	± 11	0	14	7	± 10
Malleostapediopexy (n = 58)	-8	53	16	± 13	0	45	18	± 9
Incudoplatinopexy or incudovestibulopexy (n = 7)	8	41	15	± 6	5	22	14	± 6
Malleoplatinopexy or malleovestibulopexy (n = 11)	2	38	18	± 14	0	47	18	± 14

As was already mentioned, *Kley* [248] and *Glaninger* [139] had recommended to wait with ossicular-chain reconstruction until the immediate sequelae of the trauma had subsided. The findings presented in chapters 3.4.6 and 3.4.10, on the other hand, indicated that the results after the repair of a ruptured TM are the better the earlier surgery is undertaken. It was therefore of interest to examine the correlation of the audiometric results with the interval between trauma and surgery in the present series. An analysis of this kind could only be carried out in a group of patients that was sufficiently large but also sufficiently homogeneous so that the results would not be influenced by single aberrant results and by other factors, the surgical method, for example. The group of malleostapediopexies, carried out with the aid of either autologous or homologous incudes, appeared suitable from this standpoint: the surgical technique had been sufficiently uniform; the results did not vary too widely, and the group (58 patients) was the only one of sufficient size. The time was subdivided into four periods that were deliberately made unequal in length: 0–6 weeks, the time period of the hemotympanum [377]; 7 weeks to 6 months, the time period of spontaneous repair [139, 248]; 7 months to 3 years, the time period of early surgery, undertaken after the ME lesion had healed, and more than 3 years, the time period of late surgery.

Table LI presents the results of this survey, indicating that the audiometric results improved continuously over the first three time periods, while the conductive impairment remaing after surgery decreased. During the period of late surgery, there was still a noticeable audiometric gain, but the remaining conductive impairment had once more become larger. However, none of the differences are statistically significant. Therefore, the results of table LI

Table LI. Audiometric results after interpositioning of the incus: role of the interval between trauma and surgery

Internal between trauma and surgery	Auditory gain (dB) ± 1 SD	Remaining conductive loss (dB) ± 1 SD
0–6 weeks (n = 9)	10.3 ± 6.6	20.4 ± 10.8
7 weeks to 6 months (n = 4)	12.5 ± 5.4	19.0 ± 4.0
7 months to 3 years (n = 14)	13.9 ± 8.3	14.8 ± 7.1
> 3 years (n = 25)	15.2 ± 12.7	18.7 ± 10.6

may only be taken as indicating a possible trend: i.e. when in doubt, one may wait for at least 6 months before carrying out surgery for the improvement of hearing.

No explanations can be given for the time dependence of the results presented in table LI. One may only speculate: shortly after an injury, there may still be mucous membrane lesions and sanguineous extravasates present in the ME, inviting formation of scars and adhesions that may impair the mobility of the ossicular chain and thus reduce the transmission of sound.

4.6. Discussion of Surgical Results

Ossicular-chain injuries were caused most frequently, i.e. in 75% of the documented cases by blunt skull traumata, and they occurred in 23% of all TB fractures. Traffic accidents were the dominant precipitating cause. With respect to TM perforations, as will be recalled, traffic accidents played only a minor role (cf. chapter 3.4.1). It appears, however, that the increasing motorization rendered ossicular-chain defects of the type under discussion more frequent. The improved chances of patient survival brought about by modern emergency measures might also contribute to the fact that traumatically induced ossicular-chain lesions are more frequently encountered clinically [224]. Ossicular- chain defects without simultaneous TB fractures were also seen after blunt skull trauma, but not very frequently. One may safely assume that a conductive impairment results from an ossicular-chain lesion in about 2% of all blunt skull traumata. That is a higher frequency than that reported by earlier authors [65, 139].

Young males between the ages of 11 and 30 years were most frequently involved in traffic accidents. Skull traumata caused by falling and by being hit were also prevailing among males, but in the ages between 20 and 50 years.

Compared to blunt skull traumata, other causes of ossicular-chain lesions played only minor roles. Second in frequency were iatrogenic injuries, most of them incurred during simple mastoidectomies. They constituted 13% of the total. Third in frequency were blast traumata, caused, for example, by explosions. (Also included in this group were two stapedial fractures produced by slaps in the face.) Direct transtympanal injuries were quite rarely seen, i.e. in only 3 cases (2%). The most likely reason for this finding was that these injuries only infrequently involve the posterosuperior quadrant. (In our own material, there were only 13 such cases out of a total of 66, i.e.

20%; cf. chapter 3.4.3.) As was already mentioned, incus and stapes are apparently protected to some degree by the protruding posterior wall of the EEC. If penetrating the posterosuperior quadrant at all, an instrument usually enters the ME between the mallar handle and the long incudal crus. And then again, one should also think of the possibility that an intruding foreign body might simply push the TM into the tympanic cavity. The resulting excessive displacement of the malleus could be sufficient to interrupt the ossicular chain. However, we have not encountered any such cases. The resistance of the ossicular joints against their disruption is apparently suprior to that of the TM against its perforation. In the 3 patients with direct mechanical ossicular-chain injuries, the TM had apparently been perforated in the posterosuperior quadrant, since there were scars in this region.

The mechanism underlying direct mechanical injuries of the ossicular chain appears to be well understood. However, that is not the case with such injuries caused by blunt skull trauma. That they are produced *indirectly* by forces striking the skull (which is contrary to *Ulrich*'s [443] earlier notion of 1926) hardly needs any further discussion. *Hough* [202] saw three potential causes for ossicular lesions of this kind: (1) tetanic contractions of the middle-ear muscles; (2) vibratory impulses that, traveling through the skull, are being transmitted to the ossicles, and (3) ossicular inertia that should come into play on sudden accelerations and decelerations of the skull produced by an impact.

The present results do not permit to render a constructive comment to the above item 1. *Kley* [248], for one, held this kind of origin for highly improbable. With regard to item 2, *Dürrer* et al. [87] were able to show that the magnitudes of vibratory deformations of the skull produced by a trauma decrease fast from the point of input in all directions of travel; at a distance of only a few centimeters they can hardly be recorded anymore. It is not very likely that pressure waves could be transmitted in this manner to the ossicles in magnitudes sufficient for their luxation or fracture, especially since the ossicles are not in firm contact with the bones of the skull.

At first thought, it seems that a sudden acceleration might be capable of jerking the incus out of position, especially since it is only suspended by its ligaments and joints. However, the ossicular masses are so small that the forces generated by such accelerations must likewise be small. The mass of the incus is usually given as 54 mg [351, 428].

On may calculate the acceleration required for the disruption of the incudostapedial joint on the basis of the resistance against its interruption as determined by *Glaninger* [138] (which he expressed in terms of the force needed to just disrupt the joint). Taking his value of 52 g and the incudal mass as 54 mg, one obtains an acceleration value a:

$$a = 10^4 m \times s^{-2}.$$

To approach this value, a skull had to be stopped within 1 msec from an impact velocity of 36 km/h (corresponding to a fall from a height of 5 m). Considering the elastic deformability of the osseous skull and the plasticity of the covering soft tissues, one should not even consider a deceleration of such magnitude. Crash tests on dummies with an impact velocity of 50 km/h (as generated for example after a fall from a height of 9.6 m) produced 'mere' decelerations of $1.5–2 \times 10^3$ m $\times$ s^{-2} (W. Hoechtl, Research Department, VW factory, Wolfsburg, FRG, personal communication, 1980). A disruption of the ossicular chain due to the inertia of its members could therefore not occur until the skull is stopped quite suddenly from considerably higher impact velocities. This should produce skull injuries that are not compatible with continued life. Hence, from a practical standpoint, the inertia hypothesis of Hough [202] concerning the origin of ossicular defects can hardly be supported.

The experimental studies of Guerrier [158] appear to be considerably more relevant from the present standpoint. (They had already been briefly described in chapter 3.5 with respect to the production of TM perforations by blunt skull traumata.) Guerrier saw deformations of the skull produced by an impact as the main cause of ossicular defects. That the cranial skull may be elastically deformed is well known [294, 295, 452]. With the aid of improved methods of measurement, Guerrier et al. [160, 161, 163] were able to demonstrate that, following a lateral impact, the walls of the tympanic cavity are deformed, i.e. the tegmen tympani moves down and the lateral attic wall sideways. Guerrier assumed that the downward movement of the tegmen tympani might push the incus in a caudal direction. (In extreme cases, fragments of the tegmen tympani may be thrown into the cavity or myelomeningoceles made to prolapse into it.) Such deformations should lead to the luxation of the incus or, when the incudal joints remain intact, to a shearing displacement of the stapedial crura relative to the footplate [428].

The sideways displacement of the lateral attic wall, likewise observed by Guerrier et al. [160], might widen the tympanic cavity in the transversal direction. Its effect is demonstrated by the clinical finding that most longitudinal fractures run across the tegmen tympani from posterolaterally to anteromedially (cf. chapter 5, later on). This would indicate that tension was introduced in a direction normal to that of the fracture. Moreover, the compression of the tympanic annulus ought to lead to an elliptical deformation of the TM [36], as was already mentioned in the discussion of TM ruptures (cf. chapter 3.5). This in turn ought to make the cone of the TM shallower and hence move the malleus handle laterally. The malleus should pull the incus along and this would stress, and eventually luxate, the incudostapedial joint as was actually observed in animal studies [187].

These are of course only hypothetical considerations, although they are based on well-established findings. In the following a clinical case will be briefly described that supports the present hypothesis quite well:

Patient R.J., female, 46 years; brain concussion during a car accident; longitudial fracture of the right temporal bone and CSF discharge from the right ear that ceased spontaneously. Otological examination 9 months after the accident because of persistent complaints of vertigo. Clinical findings: TM intact, tangible step in the posterosuperior portion of the osseus canal wall. High-frequency hearing loss together with a conductive component of 10 dB in the right ear, positive stapedial reflex. Evoked nystagmus was beating toward the right, although both ears were equally excitable by caloric stimulation. Explorative tympanotomy because of the suspicion of a perilymphatic fistula. Surgical findings: 'healed' luxation of the incudostapedial joint that is held together by scar tissue. Chorda tympani lying *medially* to the long incudal crus. Vertical fissures in the horizontal portion of the facial nerve canal and in the promontory on either side of the OW niche. Annular ligament torn in its anterior region, perilymphatic fistula and fracture of the footplate rim in the same region. The fistula was covered with connective tissue and mucous membrane and the incus transposed. Some postsurgical audiometric gain (remaining conductive loss of 5 dB; sensorineural component unchanged). Vertigo still persisting. Surgical revision after 4 months: the perilymphatic fistula was still patent, the footplate fragment floating free. The latter was removed. The fistula was once more covered. Postoperative improvement of the vertigo.

The case under discussion presents a number of different points:

(1) The chorda tympani could have only reached the medial side of the incus if the incudostapedial joint had become temporarily disrupted. However, this could not have been brought about by a movement of the incus in the caudal direction, which would have simply placed the chorda deeper into the angle between malleus and incus. Rather, it ought to have been produced by the kind of lateral displacement of the incus just described.

(2) At the occasion of both operations, i.e. 9 and 13 months after the trauma, the fractured footplate showed no tendency to heal. Even at the time

of the second operation, the footplate fragment was still floating freely in the OW.

(3) In spite of the fissures in the osseous labyrinthine capsule visible in the region of the promontory, the cochlear function was rather well preserved; there was only a moderate high-tone loss. A similar finding was described earlier [372], although in the latter case the vestibular function was abolished.

(4) The spontaneous stoppage of the CSF discharge will be further discussed in chapter 5.2 and the existence of the perilymphatic fistula and its symptomatology in chapter 7.

The present study confirms some other recent reports [19, 56, 139, 203, 249] on the types of ossicular defects and their sites. *Luxations* were the most frequent ossicular injuries and, among them, those of the incudostapedial joint were leading, followed by those of the incudomallar joint. Ossicular *fractures* were only rarely seen, relatively most frequent among them being those of the stapedial crura, followed by those of the mallar handle. Osseous *fixations* occurred even less frequently [287]. Their formation appeared to depend on the local situation (bony fragments, mucous membrane lesions) and also on the time elapsed after the original trauma. A bony fixation of the footplate was seen only once, which is in contrast to the findings of *Charachon* et al. [58], who considered this a frequent form of injury. An ossicular defect in the presence of an otosclerotic stapes fixation was also observed once (in a postmortem specimen). With 136 cases confirmed during surgery and 7 more during postmortem examination, this amounts to an incidence of only 0.7%. Hence, this combination was not found more frequently than what should be expected on the basis of the general occurrence of otosclerotic stapes fixation, usually given as about 1% [e.g. 24]. An increase of ossicular lesions in the presence of otosclerosis, as claimed by several authors [213, 322, 346, 362], could therefore not be demonstrated.

The most important criteria for arousing one's suspicion that an ossicular defect may in fact exist are patient's history and the pure-tone audiometric results. The otoscopic examination fails to give positive indications in more than 50% of all blunt skull traumata and in about 6% of transtympanal, ossicular-chain injuries. The notion of some authors [81, 92, 395, 444], i.e. that the presence of a Carhart notch would confirm the diagnosis of otosclerosis and exclude a traumatic ossicular lesion, was shown to be faulty: In the present series, 11% of the presurgical audiograms revealed a Carhart notch which, in about one third of them, could no longer be demonstrated after surgery. In 23% of cases, the result of impedance testing appeared not to agree with the findings made during surgery. Moreover, 3 of 7 tympanograms did not give any indication concerning the type of lesion eventually found.

When in doubt, i.e. on the mere suspicion that an ossicular lesion might exist, one should perform an exploratory tympanotomy [81, 163], even if one or several of the aforementioned diagnostic criteria are missing.

If the conductive component of the hearing loss present is larger than 20 dB and the Rinne test negative, surgery is indicated since, with a high degree of probability, one may expect to achieve a useful audiometric gain.

Firm guidelines for the choice of the *method* most suitable for ME reconstruction cannot be presented because of the large variability of ossicular lesions and the large number of surgical techniques at one's disposal. It appears that surgical reposition, mobilization and, if implants are required, the use of stiff, biologically inert material (ceramic or wire) produce optimal results. Statistically, however, this statement cannot be corroborated.

The same goes for the choice of *timing*. One gains the impression that results turn out best when surgery is performed between the sixth month and the third year after the injury, as was already suggested by *Kley* [248]. Statistically, however, this cannot be proven either. It is understood that early surgery is required if any otogenic complication is imminent or if a perilymphatic fistula is present.

5. Fractures of the Temporal Bone and Their Complications

A complete review of injuries to the lateral skull base would far exceed the scope of the present monograph. On the other hand, as was already mentioned in relation to TM injuries (chapter 3), laterobasal skull fractures usually involve the ME in a variety of ways. Therefore, a brief, general review of TB fractures is needed before we are able to proceed with a discussion of the different forms of ME lesions caused by them.

Ever since the publication of the classical papers by *Messerer* [294, 295] and *von Wahl* [452], skull fractures are divided in linear and depressed fractures, according to their mode of origin.

The definition of *linear fractures* is clear. They are usually produced when the skull bones are subjected to strong bending forces. (This mode of injury will be described in some detail later on in the present chapter.)

Depressed fractures are produced by forces acting on circumscribed areas with local infraction or penetration of the skull bones (e.g. the pressure-activated bolt in *Messerer*'s [295] 1884 experiments). Fissures and fracture lines may radiate away from the place of impact [452]. Injuries of that kind rarely involve the osseous walls of the ME, which is protected by its position deep in the temporal bone. Only two injuries of the ear, possibly produced in this manner, were reported in the literature: (a) a fracture of the anterior wall of the osseous EEC following either a fall onto the chin or a direct impact, whereby the mandibular capitulum was driven deep into the mandibular fossa [153, 216], and (b) another fracture caused by an instrument entering via the EEC, penetrating the ME and destroying part of its medial wall. Based on his own cadaver experiments, *Zaufal* [475–477] thought it possible that the carotid artery could be injured in this manner. *Schwartze* [382] was the first to desribe the clinical findings in a patient: a knitting needle had penetrated the TM and the tegmen tympani. The accident was immediately followed by discharge of CSF from the ear and, some time later, by a meningitis. From the literature, *Rothman* et al. [363] collected 9 cases of fractures produced via the EEC, adding a tenth case of their own. All of them involved the Fallopian canal and resulted in FN paralyses. TM injuries caused by foreign bodies entering via the EEC are quite common (cf. chapter 3.1.1). Less frequent are ossicular injuries produced in this manner (cf. chapter 4.5.1) and least frequent fractures of the ME walls.

By definition, gunshot injuries belong into the class of depressed fractures, since the incident force acts on a small circumscribed area. As discussed in the monographs of *Haymann* [177–181] and of *Mündnich* [318], the mode of injury is rather complex, since the bullet is usually deflected from its straight course by the skull bones and since additional injuries are produced by the increase in intracranial pressure. As our own collection hardly contains any gunshot injuries, this special form of skull trauma will not be discussed further in the present monograph.

The majority of skull fractures involving the ME are those of the lateral skull basis in the region of the TB. *Messerer* [294, 295] and *von Wahl* [452] demonstrated experimentally that a human skull firmly mounted between two points of support will be elastically deformed when being compressed. When its elastic limits are exceeded, it breaks where the stress was largest, i.e. at the place of maximal displacement. These are referred to as indirect or 'bursting' fractures. *Von Wahl* [452] and *Hermann* [190] were able to demonstrate that, as the rule, the region of largest stress is at the base of the skull and that the fracture lines extend in the direction of the impact. With respect to the lateral skull basis, this means that forces acting in the *temporal* region ought to induce fractures running *parallel* to the axis of the TB and that those acting in the *occipital* region ought to induce fractures running *transversally* to that axis. *Barnick* [20] was the first to examine the effects of such fractures on the auditory organ in postmortem specimens. His results together with those of *Sakai* [369] as well as others, who had conducted histological studies [262, 442, 443], showed that most fracture lines can be reduced to a few typical courses. (They will be described later in the present chapter.) These conclusions were later confirmed in clinical studies [38, 249, 450].

Longitudinal TB fractures run typically from the squama along the posterosuperior wall of the EEC. After breaking the 'bridge', they continue going forward through the tegmen tympani, either in front or behind the incudomallar joint. In the region of the geniculate ganglion, they run medially *around* the labyrinth, which remains intact. From here, the fracture lines pass along the roof of the Eustachian canal or that of the carotid canal, and then along the anterior margin of the petrous pyramid, to end in the foramen lacerum. They may, however, continue into the sphenoidal bone and thus toward the opposite side. *Kley* [248] mentioned that such fractures occasionally enter the EEC from above or, when coming from the squama, immediately enter the tegmen tympani.

As was already mentioned in the discussion of ossicular luxations (cf. chapter 4.6), TB fractures may initially be distended to quite some extent, depending on the force(s) producing them, so that their osseous rims are temporarily split apart. *Helms* [189] was able to demonstrate such temporary dehiscences, while studying experimentally produced longitudinal TB fractures with the aid of high-speed motion pictures.

Transversal fractures, as a rule, take their origin in the posterior fossa. They pass through the petrous pyramid either in the region of the internal auditory canal (*inner*, transversal fractures [450]), thereby injuring the nerves contained in it as well as the cochlea; or they fracture the labyrinth itself, emerging on the surface of the medial wall of the ME between the two windows. In this manner, the vestibular portion of the labyrinth may be separated from the cochlear portion (*outer*, transversal fractures [450]). *Grove* [153] pointed out that the region between the two windows is a preferred location of fissures in the labyrinthine capsule. This had already been observed by *Barnick* [20] in a postmortem specimen. He found such fissures, *without penetrating fractures*, but even then the cochlear function was abolished. *Schlittler* [372] described a similar case; however, the function of the inner ear was at least partially preserved.

Most authors do not believe that the tympanic annulus can be fractured by itself. They see such infractions as tangible evidence of longitudinal fractures [e.g. 262]. *Voss* [450] considered the blow-off fracture of the mastoid process a special form.

Numerically, the longitudinal fractures exceed the transversal ones by a wide margin. *Boenninghaus* [38] and *Tos* [436, 438] found a percentage ratio of 90:10 in favor of the longitudinal fractures among 86 or 248 TB fractures, respectively. *Voss* [450] saw 46 longitudinal fractures, 6 transversal and 6 combined ones. For his material, *Grove* [153, 154] gave a ratio of 146:8:8. *Kley* [249] collected 493 longitudinal fractures from the literature, but found only 62 transversal and 22 combined ones, i.e. ratios of 85:11:4. Longitudinal fractures are said to be prevalent in well-pneumatized mastoids and transversal fractures in poorly pneumatized ones [461]. The two types of fractures may also occur in combination.

To demonstrate and classify TB fractures in postmortem specimens is a rather straightforward task. Clinically, however, this is much more difficult, which accounts for the fact that different authors weigh the various signs and symptoms in a different manner.

A blunt skull trauma that fractures the skull basis simultaneously represents a closed brain injury. *Hough* [202], on the basis of his analysis of 31
cases of ME injuries, postulated that they should, without exception, be
accompanied by loss of consciousness and bleeding from the ear. (There was
no explicit mention of TB fractures.) Among 211 patients with TB fractures,
however, *Grove* [153, 154] found 28 (13%), in whom no loss of consciousness had occurred at the time of the injury. *Boenninghaus* [38] found no
signs or symptoms of a brain concussion in 48 cases (27%) of a total group
of 175 patients with frontobasal or laterobasal skull fractures. *Tos* [436, 438]
saw 230 patients with TB fractures of traumatic origin. In 9% of them, there
were neither signs of endocranial complications nor evidence of any additional fractures. *Gros* [152] stated that one should not draw any conclusions
as regards the seriousness of the accompanying ear injury on the basis of the
gravity of the skull-brain trauma.

The situation is similar with *Hough*'s second criterion, bleeding from
the ear. *Boenninghaus* [38] as well as *Kley* [249] maintained that, in the case
of longitudinal TB fractures, the TM is almost invariably torn and that it is
this injury that causes varying degrees of bleeding from the ear. And then
again, *Lange* [262] had already found that the TM may remain intact in
cases of longitudinal fractures extending into the external canal. Yet, there
may still be bleeding from the ear, i.e. when the canal skin over the fracture
is torn [352]. Clinical reports variously give the relative incidence of bleeding
from the ear in patients with longitudinal TB fractures as 32% [450], 69%
[154], 42% [352], and 76% [361].

In a group of 222 longitudinal TB fractures, *Tos* [436, 438] found TM
ruptures and bleeding from the involved ear in 58%; bleeding in the presence
of a hemotympanum, but with the TM intact, in 17%; no traces of blood in
the ear canal, but a hemotympanum behind an intact TM, in 23% and,
finally, no blood on either side of an intact TM in 2% of his patients.

Grove [153, 154] as well as *Guerrier* et al. [163] considered subperiosteal
bleeding, which manifests itself as a hematoma over the mastoid within the
first week after the injury, a diagnostically important indication of longitudinal fractures. (This is also known as the 'sign of Battle' [352].) *Voss* [450]
as well as *Boenninghaus* [38], on the other hand, regarded such hematomata
as evidence of ruptured sigmoid sinus.

In most cases, there is relatively little bleeding from the EEC. If there is
any, it may stem from the torn skin of the EEC, from ruptured TM or from
lesions of the ME mucosa. Bleeding may only become serious when larger
blood vessels are lacerated, such as the sigmoid sinus [38] or the middle

meningeal artery [450]. Simultaneous bleeding from nose and mouth indicates that the fracture extends into the sphenoid [352]. If the carotid artery is also injured (in approximately 1% of cases [249]), patients will soon exsanguinate [154]. In some such cases, it is possible to prevent death by ligating the carotid at a suitable place [389] or by covering the tear with a balloon catheter [67, 320, 394]. Bleeding around the ear, either from the EEC or in the form of a mastoid hematoma or a hemotympanum, is an important sign of a longitudinal fracture. However, it is not present in every case [436]. Moreover, it may occur in the *absence* of a TB fracture, for example, when the soft tissues of the EEC are lacerated by a fragmentation of the socket of the temperomandibular joint [154] or when only the TM is ruptured [352].

With *transversal* TB fractures, the tympanic annulus and the TM usually remain intact. Therefore, one should not expect any bleeding from the ear. Nevertheless, if the fracture extends into the medial wall of the ME, the mucosa may be injured and, consequently, there may be a hemotympanum. *Voss* [450] found a hemotympanum in 8 out of a group of 104 transversal fractures. *Grove* [153, 154] likewise saw 8 hematomata, without mentioning if these had occurred in patients with transversal fractures, of which he saw 16 in his group of 211 TB fractures. *Tos* [436, 438] found hemotympana in 5 of 11 purely transversal fractures. *Kley* [249] considers it a frequent, but not a mandatory, sign of a transversal fracture. *Boenninghaus* [40] stated that it is almost always present. However, neither of the two last-named authors presented any data.

A dehiscence in the osseous canal wall caused by a longitudinal TB fracture is usually covered by swollen soft tissues and blood coagula as long as the injury is fresh. After the local lacerations have healed, otoscopic examination often reveals a step, or a small gap, in the posterior wall of the osseous canal. This is considered firm evidence for a longitudinal fracture, which is said to occur in 50% of all cases [99]. If there was a TM injury, it has usually healed by this time and can no longer be discerned [437]. Otoscopic examination of patients with transversal fractures at such a late time does not provide any useful, additional information.

In addition to patient's history and the results of the otoscopic examination, functional tests may provide important clues about TB fractures and their location. Longitudinal fractures usually bypass the labyrinth without injuring it. However, they almost invariably involve the ME structures producing a hemotympanum and possibly an ossicular defect, as was already mentioned. A conductive hearing impairment can therefore be demonstrated in nearly every case [249]. *Tos* [436, 438] found hearing losses smaller than 20 dB in 24% of his patients. *Escher* [100–102] mentioned conductive impairments in 23 out of 33 patients with longitudinal fractures. (However, it is not clear if these were found at the occasion of an early examination.) In a group of 25 patients with longitudinal fractures, *Proctor* et al. [352] saw 9 patients with purely sensorineural losses, 13 with combined hearing losses, and 3 with normal hearing. *Grove* [153, 154] found hearing losses in 65% of 180 patients with longitudinal fractures he had examined, but he did not differentiate conductive losses from sensorineural ones. In a group of 72 patients with longitudinal fractures, *Boenninghaus* [38] encountered conductive impairments in 60 of them (83%). After the hemotympanum has subsided, i.e. within 4–6 weeks [377, 437], the conductive impairment also diminishes, except in those patients in whom the ossicular chain is interrupted, as was already discussed in chapter 4.

Even in the presence of a purely longitudinal fracture, a cochlear impairment may exist, either in the form of a high tone loss (type II of *Escher* [99]) or in the form of a flat cochlear loss (type III of *Escher* [99]). Several authors [250, 442, 450] saw microfissures of the labyrinthine capsule as the cause of such cochlear lesions; others [262, 266, 415, 443] thought that they were caused by bleeding into the inner-ear spaces; still others [20, 365, 467] that fluid pressure pulses, produced by the impact, might directly damage the inner-ear structures ('labyrinthine concussion'). *Fleischer* [118] as well as *von Ilberg* [208] were of the opinion that there is no uniform pathology, but that all three forms of damage might occur. In his statistic on 222 longitudinal fractures, *Tos* [436, 438] gave the incidence of apparent inner-ear damage as follows: moderate high-tone losses, up to 25 dB, in 21%, severe high-tone losses in 6%, and total cochlear losses in 4%. Corresponding figures of *Boenninghaus* [38] are: moderate sensorineural losses in 19%, severe ones in 10%, and total cochlear losses in 8% of 72 patients with longitudinal fractures. *Proctor* et al. [352] found cochlear impairments in 22 of 25 patients (=88%). *Schuknecht* [377] expressed the opinion that some cochlear damage — at least in the form of a 4-kHz notch — is present in nearly every case of a longitudinal fracture. *Proctor* et al. [352] mentioned the existence of tinnitus as an additional sign of cochlear damage in 7 out of 28 patients with longitudinal TB fractures, i.e. in 25%.

In contrast to the longitudinal fractures, *transverse* fractures run either across the internal meatus or pass directly through the labyrinth, as was already mentioned (inner and outer fractures of *Voss* [450]). They are therefore responsible for severe injuries of the labyrinthine structures and/or the

8th nerve. As a rule, the involved ear is rendered completely deaf [38, 153, 249, 352, 450]. There are only a few reports about partially preserved cochlear functions [e.g. 372].

In cases of longitudinal fractures, the *vestibular* function is similarly impaired. Moreover, it is often difficult to differentiate peripheral vestibular lesions from central lesions that are caused by the skull-brain trauma [38, 249, 352]. If impairments of the vestibular organs can be demonstrated, cochlear functions, almost invariably, are also impaired. *Boenninghaus* [38] found 15 patients with peripheral vestibular lesions among 86 patients with laterobasal fractures (including 6 transversal fractures, which were not listed separately as such); 11 of these patients were completely deaf in the involved ear and 2 others had a cochlear hearing impairment. In 2 of the 15, there was nothing but vestibular hypoexcitability; after some time, the function recovered fully in both patients. *Proctor* et al. [352] found caloric inexcitability in 4 patients out of 26 with longitudinal fractures. 7 of these patients displayed spontaneous nystagmus. 2 of them were completely deaf in the involved ear, owing to combined longitudinal and transversal fractures. In 2 others, there was a high-tone hearing loss. *Grove* [153, 154] found vestibular disturbances, which he did not specify in detail, in about 75% of all longitudinal and transversal fractures. *Hough* [203] mentioned the occurrence of spells of vertigo in 13% of his 31 patients with longitudinal fractures.

With *transversal* fractures and concomitant destruction of the inner ear and/or the 8th nerve, vestibular function, as a rule, is also severely impaired, i.e. there is vertigo, spontaneous nystagmus and the ears involved are calorically not excitable [38, 249, 450]. Nevertheless, cases with partially preserved vestibular function, but completely abolished cochlear function, have been described more frequently than the reverse combination ([250] 2 cases; [153] 3 cases; see also [252]). These findings once more confirm the classical rule that the vestibular organs are more resistant against trauma than the cochlea.

The fourth important diagnostic point in cases of TB fractures is the X-ray examination, but its value is disputed. It is the consensus of opinion that routine lateral-skull X-ray pictures rarely permit demonstration of a fracture line in the complex structures of the skull basis [35, 38, 249]. *Blohmke* [35], however, expressed the opinion that fracture lines can *always* be demonstrated in the projections of *Stenvers, Schüller* and *Mayer. Gros* [152] also held these projections sufficient for making the diagnosis of a fracture, but gave no figures. *Boenninghaus* [38] thought this only possible when there is a sufficiently wide osseous dehiscence and when the X-ray beam meets it at right angles. In his opinion, X-ray pictures do not provide the correct diagnosis in more than 80% of all cases. *Grove* [153, 154] was able to demonstrate only a few transversal fractures by X-rays and longitudinal fractures only when they radiated into the cranial vault. Table LII presents a summary, collected from the literature, on the value of X-ray diagnosis in cases of suspected TB fractures. (In table LII, the projections of *Stenvers, Schüller, Mayer, Altschul-Uffenorde, Runstroem II, Chausse* and others are considered 'survey' pictures.) The possibility of obtaining a correct diagnosis of TB fractures from X-ray pictures, as indicated by the numbers presented in table LII, differ widely, and the recommendations for its use vary accordingly.

Samuel [370] as well as *Bollaert* et al. [42] considered *tomography* indispensable for a proper diagnosis. *Roche* [360] acknowledged the value of tomography, but he wanted its use restricted to special cases, because of its large technical requirements and the high X-ray dosage needed. *Terrahe* [429] suggested to use a series of transorbital X-ray pictures, the angle being changed by 3° from one picture to the next. He considered tomography necessary only for the verification of ossicular discontinuities and in some special cases, i.e. when the exact course of a fracture line is to be ascertained. Although they recognized the high value of tomography for the diagnosis of

Table LII. Temporal bone fractures: the value of roentgenological examinations (literature survey; percentages given in parentheses)

Author	Longitudinal fractures			Transversal fractures		
	number of cases	positive results		number of cases	positive results	
		standard X-ray pictures	tomograms		standard X-ray pictures	tomography
Müller and Edel [317]	37	21 (57)	–	12	6 (50)	11 (91)
Proctor et al. [352]	28	18 (64)	–	16	8 (50)	–
Roche [360]	16	7 (44)	14 (88)	16	8 (50)	16 (100)
Tos [437]	222	110 (50)	–	26	(69)	–
	Combined longitudinal and transversal fractures					
Boenninghaus [39]	–	(80)	–			
Guerrier et al. [163]	130	57 (44)	–			
Rohrt [361]	120	(86)	–			
Voss [450]	38	(63)				

transversal fractures, *Müller and Edel* [317] were quite sceptical, since they personally were able to detect 8 out of 10 *longitudinal* fractures simply in survey pictures; tomography, in their experience, did not provide any additional information. In 1 case, it had missed a longitudinal fracture that was later found surgically; it was in only 1 case of theirs that tomography alone secured the diagnosis.

Boenninghaus [38] cautioned against false-positive diagnoses of fractures in the evaluation of X-ray pictures, which may be due to a wrong interpretation of osseous sutures and vascular grooves; but he gave no figures about the incidence of such faulty diagnoses.

Summarizing at this point, one may state that in many cases the findings made by otoscopic, functional and X-ray examinations do not always agree. Hence, the diagnosis of TB fractures must often rest on only two, or even one, of these measures. It is highly questionable if the combination of posttraumatic deafness and loss of vestibular function alone support the diagnosis of a transversal fracture when there was never a hemotympanum and no positive X-ray finding were made either. Complications that will be discussed below may sometimes provide additional diagnostic clues.

Uncomplicated TB fractures do not require any therapy. As a rule, the fracture is not stressed mechanically and it must therefore not necessarily be put 'in splints'. On the other hand, it is most likely the very lack of a mechanical stress that is responsible for the fact that callus is not being formed [38]. Especially fractures of the labyrinthine capsule show no tendency to heal. The enchondral bone, which constitutes the thickest layer, forms no callus at all and the endosteal and periosteal layers that are able to do so are relatively thin [153]. Most of these fractures are held together by connective-tissue scars [324, 378, 443]. In a case published by *Manasse* [286], the fracture lines present in the labyrinthine capsule and in the stapes footplate showed no osseous union, 15 years after the original trauma. Nevertheless, sometimes there is excessive ossification, which may obliterate the entire labyrinth ('periosteitis ossificans' [247, 286]).

Until the first decade of the present century, *therapy* was confined to the management of the brain trauma that was simultaneously present. *Linck* [266] and *Voss* [449] pointed out that a TB fracture must be regarded as an *open* skull trauma on account of the communication of the endocranium with the pneumatic spaces of the ME or even with the EEC. They considered active intervention mandatory because of the potential invasion by pathogenic organisms. *Voss* [450], in particular, postulated that every TB fracture requires surgical revision of the ME spaces, either for therapeutic reasons, i.e.

to eradicate a reservoir of pathogenic organisms if an endocranial infection had already taken place, or for preventive reasons, i.e. to close a potential port of entry for such organisms. There is hardly any doubt that this recommendation opened the way to an active management of skull-base fractures on the part of the otosurgeon, an area that up to that time had been considered the exclusive domain of the general surgeon. However, the introduction of antibiotics permitted the abandonment of the rigorous preventive regime. In cases of uncomplicated TB fractures, the currently accepted rule is to establish an exact diagnosis, to follow the patient carefully, and to simply wait for possible complications [38, 99, 249]. The ear canal should not be cleansed, especially not irrigated, when there had been any bleeding. Only *Guerrier* et al. [163] advocated to drain a hemotympanum by means of a myringotomy. More recently, a reconstructive indication has been added to the therapeutic ones [99]. In addition to the management of injuries of the TM and of the ossicular chain that were already discussed, this includes the surgical repair of FN lesions (cf. chapter 5.4.4).

Boenninghaus [38] and *Kley* [249] both called for surgical intervention in the cases of the following complications of TB fractures: (a) Absolute indications — dura tears; meningitis of infectious origin; open brain injury; late endocranial complications; persisting hemorrhages; life-threatening rises in endocranial pressure, and penetrating foreign bodies. (b) Relative indications — shattered fractures; widely opened ME spaces; fractures in the presence of acute or chronic ME infections and/or mastoiditis; FN lesions of traumatic origin; persisting posttraumatic conductive hearing losses, posttraumatic cholesteatoma, and posttraumatic atresias of the EEC.

(Persisting posttraumatic conductive hearing losses were already discussed in chapter 4. The last two points will be described in chapter 6. The remaining complications will be briefly discussed in the following three chapters.)

5.1. Hemorrhaging

Hemorrhages were already mentioned in the description of TB fractures. Bleeding may become very strong when either the sigmoid, the transversal sinus [249] or the middle meningeal artery [450] are injured. This may lead to considerable blood loss. The blood may enter the cranial cavity, thus compressing the brain. Bleeding from the carotid artery – possibly with formation of an arteriovenous anastomosis with the cavernous sinus – occurs only when the fracture continues into the sphenoid. Surgical management is by a transsphenoidal approach and, as such, is outside the scope of ME surgery.

Following sinus injuries, there may be other complications, besides hemorrhages, i.e. sinus thromboses (*Dixon*, cit. after [154]), air emboli, and also cerebral emboli [249].

External bleeding may be stilled temporarily by a firmly applied dressing over the ear. The fracture line, as presented in the X-ray pictures, often gives a hint with respect to the site of the hemorrhage. Angiography may be used to clarify the situation further.

Endocranial hemorrhaging is suggested by signs and symptoms of increased endocranial pressure. Required further steps to confirm the diagnosis include lumbar puncture, computer tomography and angiography.

Surgical exposure of the ME and mastoid spaces is mandatory. A bleeding vessel, when found, is ligated; a bleeding sinus is exposed and compressed; an injured transversal sinus is also ligated [249].

Grove [153, 154] reported on 7 cases of delayed hemorrhaging from the ear, up to 1 month after the trauma. He cited a communication of *Brunner*'s who stated that the most likely cause would be bleeding from a posttraumatic aneurysm of the meningeal artery. *Proctor* et al. [352], on the other hand, assumed that such late hemorrhages might originate from pathological alterations of the vascular walls in the traumatized region, brought about by infection.

5.2. Dura Injuries, Pneumatoceles and Endocranial Infections

Transverse TB fractures create an open communication between the pneumatized spaces of the ME and the fluid spaces of the inner ear. With *lateral* transversal fractures, such communications run through the medial wall of the tympanic cavity, and with *medial* fractures, through the labyrinthine capsule in the region of the musculotubal canal. These communications may also lead into the CSF space via the cochlear aqueduct. Even though this narrow channel does hardly permit any fluid exchange, it still represents a potential port of entry for infectious organisms into the endocranial space (cf. also chapter 7.4). If the sharp edges of the fracture — either longitudinal or transversal — have torn the dura, which in the region of the lateral skull basis adheres firmly to the bone [36], CSF may enter the ME, to be either discharged via a torn TM (otoliquorrhea) or to remain as fluid behind the TM (liquor-tympanum [450]). In the latter case, the fluid usually drains into the nasopharynx via the Eustachian tube [352]. (This is sometimes referred to as an oto-rhino-liquorrhea [159].) Discharge of CSF from the ear invariably points to the existence of a TB fracture. A watery fluid draining from the ear or into the nasopharynx is always supicious of being CSF. If there is also bleeding from the ear, the dressing usually shows a clear, watery ring around the central blood coagulum [249]. Synovial fluid of the jaw joint, a serous exudate of infectious origin and CSF can be differentiated from one another on the basis of their glucose content. (CSF contains about 60% glucose [40].) Intrathecally applied tracers provide definite evidence. Successfully used for this purpose were fluorescein [174] and radioactive albumin [174, 462]. Methyleneblue is said to be inadvisable, since it may produce a myelitis [174].

Not every dura lesion must necessarily lead to the discharge of CSF that manifests itself clinically. The tear in the dura may close up or it may be occluded by a brain prolapse or by pieces of brain tissue [249]. Table LIII presents a survey on the incidence of cerebrospinal discharge in cases of laterobasal fractures — longitudinal as well as transversal ones — as observed by various authors.

If one disregards the extremely high incidence reported by *Roche* [360] and if one considers the fact that in *Escher*'s patients all findings were made

Table LIII. Incidence of cerebrospinal fluid (CSF) discharge from the ear in longitudinal and transversal temporal bone fractures (literature survey)

Author	Total number of cases	Cases with CSF discharge	Percentage
Boenninghaus [38]	86	7	8
Escher [102] (limited to surgical cases)	39	5	13
Grove [153, 154]	211	8	4
Guerrier et al. [163]	130	8	6
Proctor et al. [352]	57	2	3.5
Roche [360]	32	13	40
Tos [438] (after 1 week interval)	128	7	5.5
Voss [450]	66	6	9
Piquet [345]	?	44	13 (longit. fractures) 75 (transv. fractures)

during surgery, one arrives at a clinical incidence of CSF discharge of between 3.5 and 9% in cases of TB fractures.

Discharge of air from the fractured mastoid under the periosteum was already observed by *Bezold* [31]. He referred to it as a subperiosteal pneumatocele.

That air may enter the intradural space, instead of fluid being discharged toward the outside, was first observed by *Duken* [88]. He described 2 patients in whom air had accumulated intracranially after gunshot injuries of the frontal sinus or the mastoid process, respectively. He called this an intracranial pneumatocele. *Passow* [340] was able to add to these cases 2 more collected from the literature as well as 2 of his own. In all of *Passow*'s 4 cases, however, the origin was from the paranasal sinuses. *Passow* assumed that, in these cases, the air was forced through the dura gap into the skull interior by pressure increases in the nasopharynx (pressing, blowing one's nose). *Voss* [450] described 1 pneumatocele among his 104 cases of TB fractures. Hence, an otogenic origin is apparently quite rare. *Kittel* [243] differentiated intracerebral, subdural, subarachnoidal and intraventricular pneumatoceles. (In his opinion, they should be called *pneumencephala*, since they lack the serous lining characteristic of a genuine 'cele'.) He assumed that they were brought about by a one-way valve mechanism, produced by adhesions, swollen mucous membranes or directly by the wound margins. He considered the intracranial collection of air a late complication, which may occur even after many years. Increased pressure in the pneumatic spaces, in *Kittel*'s opinion, is not a mandatory requirement for the passage of air into the intracranial spaces, since he observed an otogenic pneumatocele in the presence of a ruptured TM. According to *Kittel*, the intracerebral pneumatocele is the most frequent form (about 50% of all cases); subdural, subarachnoidal and intraventricular forms occur less frequently. Epidural pneumatoceles caused by epidural hemorrhages are least frequent, probably because the air pressure in the pneumatic spaces is not high enough to force the dura off the bone [243]. In most instances, the pneumatoceles originated from the paranasal sinuses. Only 16% of them were of otogenic origin.

The diagnosis of an intracranial pneumatocele is usually made on the basis of X-ray pictures. Clinical signs and symptoms, as a rule, are absent. When there are larger intracerebral spaces that are only partially filled with fluid, the patient or the examining physician may hear splashing noises [88]. Intracerebral pneumatoceles may also give rise to signs and symptoms of increased intracranial pressure [243].

The management of a dura defect is the same whether it manifests itself as a CSF leakage, a pneumatocele or a combination of both. If there is increased intracranial pressure, its release is mandatory [243]. In most cases, however, the air within a pneumatocele is quickly absorbed as soon as the communication is sealed [107].

It is only in rare cases that a TB fracture produces a larger gap in the tegmen tympani or in that of the antrum. If such a gap is present, a meningocele [169], an arachnoidal cyst [248] or brain tissue may prolapse into the ME (3 cases [450]; 2 cases [102]).

The gravest complication of a dura lesion in the region of the otobasis is an ascending infection, facilitated by a communication between the endocranial space and the pneumatized ME spaces, which may contain pathogenic organisms. Quite often, therefore, it leads to a meningitis. Extensively shattered fractures with sequestration and exposed necrotic brain tissue are considered to be more dangerous in this respect than smooth fractures or fissures [38].

In 486 cases with laterobasal skull fractures, the relative incidence of meningitis was 5% [149]. In a group of 104 patients with TB fractures (66 of which were operated on), *Voss* [450] found 7 cases of purulent meningitis (6.7%) — 1 of them was caused by a blow-out fracture of the tegmen tympani and the 6 others by transversal fractures. In 15 additional cases (12 longitudinal fractures and 3 transversal ones, i.e. 14% of his total), he performed surgery on the mere suspicion of a meningitis. He found meningitis to be a more frequent complication of transversal fractures than of longitudinal fractures. *Grove* [153, 154], in a survey of the literature, found an incidence of meningitis of 7–8%. He did not report figures of his own, but merely mentioned that he had found no intracranial complications in 16 patients with transversal fractures. *Boenninghaus* [38] saw meningitic complications in 6 of a total of 86 patients with TB fractures (7%); 5 of them had occurred in patients with transversal fractures (83% of the total of 6 patients). *Roche* [360] saw meningitis in 3 patients out of a total of 16 with transversal fractures (19%). The incidence was zero among 16 others with longitudinal fractures and likewise among 7 more with atypical fractures.

As a rule, the meningitis manifests itself approximately on the eighth to tenth day after the trauma [38]. In patients with longitudinal fractures, a late occurrence is quite rare. *Grove* [153, 154] described 1 such case; the symptom-free interval had been 5 months. *Fraser* (discussion remark to [325]) saw a meningitis developing a full year after a longitudinal fracture.

Following *transversal fractures*, a late onset of meningitis is more frequent (1 case after a free interval of 30 weeks [247]; 1 case after 210 days, another case after 6 months [325]; 1 case after 1 year [450]; 1 case after 2 years [38]; 1 case after 15 years [46]; and 1 case after 16 years [372]). The cause was seen in the incomplete repair of labyrinthine-capsule fractures which, as already mentioned, are only closed by connective tissue. The mucous membrane of the ME frequently forms deep pockets in these connective-tissue scars [324, 450], a condition which provides insufficient protection against ascending infections. *Voss* [450] therefore considered patients with transversal fractures as being endangered for the rest of their lives. Hence he called for preventive surgery to eradicate this potential source of a meningitis.

In cases of laterobasal skull fractures caused by blunt traumata, brain abscesses are apparently rare complications. *Grete* [149] cited 3 cases from the literature and reported 1 additional case of his own. *Voss* [450] saw a late abscess, 1.5 years after a longitudinal TB fracture. Following gunshot injuries, abscesses occur of course more often. The foreign material brought into the channel formed by the bullet and the accompanying brain injury set the condition for such a complication [38, 318, 450].

Most cases of uncomplicated dura defects do not require special therapy. 80% of them are said to close spontaneously [169]. *Escher* [100] stated that such closures take place within the first 3 days, *Tos* [439] that they may take 3 weeks. *Boenninghaus* [38] as well as *Guerrier* et al. [163], however, pointed out that the cessation of the CSF discharge frequently announces the onset of a meningitis so that this event asks for increased vigilance.

The indication for TB surgery in cases of endocranial complications, as was originally postulated by *Voss* [450] in 1936, is still valid today. Nevertheless, *Boenninghaus* [38] and *Kley* [249] suggested to restrict the preventive indication to cases with: extensively shattered fractures; those in which an injury of the dura is suspected; those with persisting CSF discharge from the ear, and those with serious ME infections (suppurative otitis media with granulations and polyps, mastoiditis and cholesteatoma). A simple posttraumatic otitis media, in their opinion, does not present an absolute indication for surgery, since it can usually be controlled by antibiotics.

Kley [249], in particular, advised the carrying out of emergency surgery only when there are life-threatening complications. Otherwise, one should administer antibiotics and wait until the patient has sufficiently recovered from his posttraumatic shock so that the surgery does not present an additional burden for him. Depending on the kind and extent of the lesion, the dura tear might be uncovered via a mastoidectomy, simple or radical as the case may require. ME pathology (mastoiditis, cholesteatoma), if present, should be taken care of, according to well-known otosurgical guidelines, followed by functional reconstruction of the ME, in accordance with tympanoplastic principles [37, 99]. The gap in the dura may be covered by a muscle or fascia transplant [38, 169, 438, 462]. When performing a radical mastoidectomy, *Boenninghaus* [38] preferred to install a cutis flap. *Fagerberg and Lodin* [107] employed lyophilized dura. *Kecht* [227] used a transtemporal approach and carried out a three-layered closure with lyophilized dura directly sown on, followed by a pedunculated muscle flap and a free bone transplant. If the inner ear is dead, *Kecht* [228] recommended a labyrinthectomy and occlusion of the ME by a fat transplant. All of these plastic closures appear to be stable. Only *Tos* [439] reported on a patient in whom the free transplant shrank twice in succession. Cerebrospinal discharge recurred both times. That a coexisting meningitis should be treated by antibiotics and a brain abscess by puncture and drainage shall only be mentioned in passing.

5.3. Facial Nerve Injuries

To discuss FN injuries under the heading of TB fractures is somewhat arbitrary, especially since fractures represent only one cause of FN palsy — and not even the most frequent one.

Cawthorne and Haynes [55] found that nearly 50% of 84 FN lesions they had encountered had been incurred during earlier ear surgery; 25 were produced by gunshots and only 16% had occurred in connection with skullbase fractures. *Jongkees* [217], similarly, found skull trauma the cause of only 25% of the 187 FN injuries he had treated surgically; 75% of them had been incurred during surgery. However, it appears that the number of FN lesions produced in this manner has decreased since the introduction of microsurgery of the ear. After conducting a literature survey, *Diamond and Frew* [73] came to the conclusion that between 1946 and 1956 FN injuries had occurred in 1.6–2% of all ears operated, but that the incidence was reduced to 0.3–0.4% in more recent times. Since there were no iatrogenic FN injuries in our own patient material that shall be presented below, this issue will not be pursued further.

Gunshot injuries occupied second place in the statistic of *Cawthorne and Haynes* [55]. They had already been mentioned by *Passow* [339] and by *Imhofer* [209]. *Passow*, in particular, pointed out that gunshots might produce FN palsies in an indirect manner, i.e. by a bullet passing close to the nerve without actually touching it. More recently, *Hooper* et al. [201]

described 6 cases of FN paralysis in a total of 8 gunshot injuries of the oto-basis. In 2 of them, the nerve was severed within its mastoid portion, and in 2 others there was a late palsy, followed by spontaneous recovery. This type of injury is mentioned only in passing, because of the lack of fresh gunshot injuries in our own material.

Finally, the intratemporal portion of the FN may be lacerated by a force acting on the tympanic portion of the nerve that hardly causes any injury to the surrounding bone; in this region, the bony shell of the Fallopian canal is rather thin and there are quite often dehiscences [76].

FN injuries produced by foreign bodies entering the tympanic cavity via the EEC were also mentioned by *Passow* [339]. *Jongkees* [217] described 2 such cases (caused by a knitting needle and a metal rod, respectively) and *Mounier-Kuhn* et al. [315] as well as *Miehlke* [298] 1 more case each. *Arora* et al. [15] reported on an FN injury produced by a twig that had penetrated the TM and entered the tympanic cavity. The TM had spontaneously healed with time. *Rothman* et al. [363] collected 9 other cases of transtympanal FN injuries from the literature and added 1 case of their own.

In addition to the mechanical injuries just described, the nerve may suffer *thermal* injuries by pieces of hot metal entering the ME ([3, 186, 298]: 1 case each). Caustic burns incurred during the treatment of some ME ailments were also described [339]. Skull traumata, even when not producing any TM injuries, may occasionally lead to FN palsies when a luxated incus is pressing on the nerve ([66, 217, 315]: 1 case each, [264]: 3 cases, [289, 290]: 4 cases). Such an effect is apparently brought about by the rebound of the lateral attic wall when it is elastically deformed by an impact on the skull.

Far more frequent than these isolated FN injuries are lesions that are produced by laterobasal skull fractures. *Diamond and Frew* [73] gave the incidence of FN palsies associated with blunt skull traumata as 1.6–4%. There is a consensus of opinion — with the exception of *Roche* [360] — i.e. that FN paralyses occur relatively much more frequently in transversal fractures than in longitudinal ones.

Table LIV, presenting absolute numbers, shows FN paralyses to be prevalent in cases with longitudinal fractures, but perhaps only because longitudinal fractures happen to be more frequent than transversal ones. In a group of 48 patients with posttraumatic FN paralyses, *Jongkees* [217] found 30 longitudinal fractures and only 5 transversal fractures. The remaining 13 fractures showed atypical courses. Yet, as was just mentioned, transversal fractures are not as frequent as longitudinal ones.

Table LIV. Incidence of longitudinal and transversal temporal bone fractures, percentages of associated facial-nerve palsies (literature survey)

Author	Total number of fractures	Ratio long./transv. fractures	Percentage of associated facial nerve palsies	
			long. fr.	transv. fr.
1 *Voss* [450]	52	9:1	18	50
2 *Grove* [153, 154]	162	9:1	19	31
3 *Proctor* et al. [352]	44	6:4	25	6
4 *Boenninghaus* [38]	86	9:1	35	38
5 *Boenninghaus* [39]	–	–	20	50
6 *Gros* [152]	–	–	30	50
7 *Hough* [203]	–	–	20	50
8 *Tos* [438]	248	9:1	15	38
9 *Roche* [360]	32	5:5	56	43
10 *Diamond and Frew* [73]	–	8:2	20	40
11 *Fisch* [116]	–	–	20	40
Total of Nos 1–4, 8, 9	624	86:14	21 (n=113)	33 (n=29)

Dietzel [79] was able to show statistically that the risk of an FN palsy occurring in conjunction with longitudinal fractures increases when the peri-labyrinthine pneumatization is extensive.

For quite some time, opinions were divided with regard to the kinds of FN injury and their locations associated with TB fractures. *Kettel* expressed the opinion (discussion remark to [217]) that they were mostly related to impairments of the blood supply to the nerve, caused by mechanical vibrations; furthermore, that direct injuries of the nerve, if and when they occurred, would take place in the mastoid portion. *Boenninghaus* [38], *Escher* [99] and *Kley* [248] concurred with this opinion. They considered the second knee of the FN the place of predilection for injuries. *Von Schulthess and Dubs* [380], in a total of 16 FN injuries associated with longitudinal TB fractures, found that 62% had indeed occurred in this region.

Earlier, *Ulrich* [443] had concluded, on the basis of his histological studies in longitudinal fractures, that FN injuries take place predominantly in the region of the geniculate ganglion. This conclusion was later endorsed by *Grove* [153, 154] and by *Proctor* et al. [352]. It was confirmed clinically during surgical exploration [79, 113, 114, 189]: In the majority of patients with FN paralyses caused by longitudinal as well as by transversal fractures, lesions of the geniculate ganglion were found in 93 or 90% of cases, respectively [114]. *Müller and Edel* [317], in a surgical and roentgenological study, found lesions of the geniculate ganglion, or lesions in the region immediately around it, in 93% of longitudinal fractures and in 70% of transversal fractures. In a study on experimental transverse fractures, *Travis* et al. [440] saw geniculate ganglion lesions in nearly every case.

Opinions are also divided about the diagnostic measures required. *Gros* [152] as well as *Diamond and Frew* [73] recommended, without qualification, to determine the place of the injury with the aid of the Schirmer test, the stapedius reflex test and gustation tests. *Jongkees* [217] held all these tests only partly reliable since, in his hands, they quite often resulted in faulty diagnoses. *Schwerdtfeger and Schwerdtfeger* [388] pointed out that, with all longitudinal fractures and with many of the transversal ones, the TM impedance test might not yield meaningful results because of the hemotympanum that is frequently present. *Miehlke and Fisch* [299] considered gustatory testing valuable for a topological diagnosis, but only under one condition, i.e. when the patient's close cooperation is assured; in patients with fresh skull traumata, that cannot be taken for granted, *Fisch* [116] regarded the Schirmer test as the only one of diagnostic significance. He held the secretion of tears to be subnormal either when the involved side secretes less than 30% of the total or when, on both sides, less than 25 mm of the filter paper is moistened within 5 min.

The difficulties involved in the roentgenological demonstration of the courses of TB fractures were already mentioned (chapter 5.0). *Krekorian* [256], as a rule, found more extensive destruction during surgery than was suggested by the X-ray findings. *Helms* [189] therefore proposed that one should not base one's decision whether to turn to surgery or not on the X-ray evidence. *Miehlke* [298] recommended to operate early if the X-ray findings indicate with certainty that the Fallopian canal is severely damaged.

Even more important than the topical diagnosis, which is based on functional and/or roentgenological findings, is the problem of the prognostic decision criteria. The relevant literature still maintains that a paresis appearing immediately after the injury suggests a nerve discontinuity and, as such, presents an unfavorable prognosis. Pareses that occur later, i.e. 4–5 days after the trauma, are thought to be produced by compressions of the nerve (due to a hematoma or an edema) or by disturbances of its blood supply; spontaneous remissions might be expected in such cases [39, 55, 298, 388].

On the other hand, it was pointed out that FN paralyses quite often cannot be diagnosed immediately after the trauma so that the time of onset remains uncertain [39]. *Jongkees* [217] voiced doubt about the value of the patient's history. In some cases, in which a free interval was claimed to have existed between the trauma and the onset of the paralysis, he found a severed nerve on surgical exploration. He was also skeptical about the spontaneous recovery of a nerve that was paralyzed late, since edema and poor blood supply might lead to axonal degeneration and scar formation and, hence, to a permanent defect. This notion was subscribed to by many other authors [39, 73, 114, 378].

Functional tests often provide rather precise prognoses. One must keep in mind, however, that the distal portion of a severed nerve is still capable of conducting impulses until the Wallerian degeneration sets in, i.e. for 3–4 days [73]. Therefore, tests for nerve excitability [55] and electroneuronography [114, 299] do not become useful until the 4-day limit has been exceeded. A decrease of excitability, requiring an increase in stimulus current of at least 3.5 mA [299], or an axonal loss of more than 90%, indicate that a permanent nerve lesion ought to be expected. During the early stages, i.e. the first 3–4 days, a complete loss of nerve function is best ascertained with the aid of electromyography [299].

Surgical intervention should have the following general aims: (a) exposure of the nerve; (b) removal of bone chips embedded in it; (c) release of the pressure caused by a hematoma or an edema, and (d) if necessary, reunification of the nerve. All these steps must be undertaken, especially when the functional tests suggested the likelihood of permanent nerve damage.

The actual approach varies with the suspected location of the nerve injury. *Ballance and Duel* [18] were the first to expose the mastoid portion of the nerve, starting at the stylomastoid foramen. *Wullstein* [471] found it preferrable to carry out a mastoidectomy first and then to search for the second knee of the FN; from this point on, he follows the nerve in a proximal direction up to the geniculate ganglion and in a distal direction down to the stylomastoid foramen. *Boenninghaus* [39] employed a similar approach. He exposed the nerve by widening the fracture line. *Krekorian* [256] used essentially the same procedure in patients with intratemporal gunshot injuries. *House and Crabtree* [205] described a transtemporal approach to the geniculate ganglion. When the nerve is found severed in the region *proximal* to the ganglion, *Miehlke* [297] advocates the Dott procedure: a craniotomy with an intracranial nerve transplantation and anastomosis to its distal portion.

The following specific steps were recommended: (a) removal of bone chips from the region of the fracture and slitting the nerve sheath open (see, however [73]); (b) in case of a discontinuity, a tension-free end-to-end anastomosis of the two stumps; (c) if required, mobilization and rerouting of the nerve, bypassing the second knee [298]; or (d) the implantation of an autologous piece of nerve into the gap, using techniques that vary little from one author to another [39, 112–114, 189, 217, 235, 236, 298, 388].

To avoid a faulty outgrowth of regenerating axons, *Fisch* [112, 116] proposed to resect the geniculate ganglion, followed by an end-to-end anastomosis of the nerve, or to clip the major superficial petrosal nerve. Many authors point to the need for an early decompression because a nerve that remains compressed for some time will degenerate; a connective tissue scar will form which impairs the axonal outgrowth [39, 114, 217, 299, 378].

Only a few figures are given in the literature about the results obtained by treating posttraumatic FN palsies:

Miehlke [298]	saw spontaneous remissions in 90% of cases, following late palsies, and in 75%, following early palsies
Boenninghaus [39]	reported 12 favorable results in 14 nerve decompressions, without giving further details
Schwerdtfeger and Schwerdtfeger [388]	reported favorable results in all patients, in whom a transtemporal decompression was performed; no particulars were given

A number of detailed reports were published [55, 116, 256, 378]. They are listed in table LV.

5.4. Our Clinical Findings

The age and sex distributions of laterobasal fractures and their causes were already presented in chapter 4.5. The analysis that follows in the present chapter considers the signs and symptoms of TB fractures and their complications only in those cases in which the course of the fracture line could be precisely documented. Precise documentation means either that the fracture was seen during surgery — in 80% of the longitudinal fractures and in 70% of the transversal ones — or that there was agreement between clinical and roentgenological findings — in 20% of the longitudinal fractures and in 30% of the transversal ones. The numbers given differ slightly from those already cited in table XXXVIII; however, a renewed listing according to age and sex would not provide any useful new information.

Table LV. Functional results after surgery of posttraumatic facial nerve palsies (literature survey; percentages given in parentheses)

Author(s)	Procedure	Results		
		good	fair	poor
Cawthorne and	decompression	31 (57)	17 (32)	6 (11)
Haynes [55]	transplant	19 (59)	8 (25)	5 (16)
(n = 86)				
Fisch [116]	decompression	(85)		
(n = 93)	end-to-end	(60)		
	anastomosis			
v. Schulthess [378]	decompression only			
(n = 17)	early palsies	5	3	1
	late palsies	4	1	1
	not known			2
	total	(52)	(24)	(24)
Krekorian [256]	autotransplants after	5 (31)	1 (31)	6 (38)
(n = 16)	gunshot injuries			

The 147 laterobasal fractures thus defined included 122 longitudinal TB fractures, 17 transversal ones and 8 with atypical courses, their percentage ratios being 83:12:5. (There was 1 patient with bilateral, longitudinal fractures.) Of the 122 *longitudinal* fractures 121 ran along the posterosuperior portion of the EEC, from there across the tegmen tympani and further on toward the geniculate ganglion or, beyond it, into the floor of the middle fossa. In only 1 patient did the fracture line traverse the mastoid, terminating behind the labyrinth, at the level of the horizontal canal.

The 17 *transversal* fractures included 7 *lateral* ones, which had split the osseous labyrinth between its cochlear and vestibular portions, and 10 *medial* ones; if surgery was performed, the latter were detected all in the region of the geniculate ganglion.

The 8 *atypical* cases included 2 with multiple fractures running along the petrous pyramid in a generally longitudinal direction; the bone was completely shattered. In both cases, the fractures were assumed to run through the labyrinth proper because vestibular *and* cochlear functions were completely abolished. Both patients displayed FN palsies. In 4 others, there were horizontal fractures of the mastoid, but they did not involve the ME. In 1 of them, the mastoid tip was completely separated from the TB, exposing the jugular bulb and the FN. In another one, the floor of the EEC was elevated by the fracture. In still another, the roof of an old radical mastoidectomy cavity was fractured and the dura torn with discharge of CSF. FN paralyses existed in all 4 patients, but neither the vestibular nor the cochlear functions were impaired.

5.4.1. Signs and Symptoms

A cerebral concussion had occurred in nearly every patient with a latero-basal fracture. In 56 patients, who were admitted to the hospital some time after the injury, this information could no longer be elicited. Of the remaining 83 patients, 77 (94%) showed signs and symptoms of a concussion. They were only missing in 5 patients with longitudinal fractures and in 1 with a transversal fracture, representing a mere 6%.

Bleeding from the involved ear was the most frequent clinical sign in the 122 patients with *longitudinal* fractures. The records of 55 patients listed varying degrees of discharge of blood from the EEC. A hemotympanum behind an intact TM was noted in 17 other patients. In 3 patients, no blood was detected, either in the EEC or in the ME. This gave a percentage ratio of 73:23:4. For the remaining 47 patients, relevant statements are missing, again mainly because they were brought to the hospital several days after the accident.

A visible step in the posterosuperior wall of the osseous part of the EEC was noted in 49 of the present patients. Discharge of CSF from the involved ear was observed in 13. In 3 of these it ceased within a week, in 1 after 1 month, in another after 4 months, and in 6 patients the time interval was unknown. 2 dura fistulae were closed surgically, 1 after 5 days and the other after 30 days. In 6 patients, a posttraumatic meningitis had made the surgical closure of the fistula mandatory (cf. chapter 5.4.3.).

7 of the 17 patients with *transversal* fractures showed bleeding from the EEC, in 2 others, there was a hemotympanum, and in 1 patient, both ME and EEC were free of blood, a ratio of 70:20:10. In the 7 remaining patients, no information was available in these respects. In no patient with a transversal fracture, nor in any patient with a longitudinal fracture, the bleeding from the ear was strong enough to warrant any therapeutic measures.

The patients with transversal fractures did of course not show any steps in the EEC walls. Discharge of CSF from the EEC occurred in 3 patients. It ceased spontaneously in 1 of them after a week, in 1 after a month and in the last patient the time interval remained undetermined. Another fistula in the region of the otobasis manifested itself 3 weeks after the trauma by discharge via the Eustachian tube. It was closed surgically and so were 2 others, after 1 week or 7 months, respectively. In 1 patient with a transversal fracture, a dura defect led to a meningitis (table LVI; cf. also chapter 5.4.3).

Impairments of inner ear functions, as might be expected, were observed more frequently in patients with transversal fractures than in those with longitudinal fractures.

Of the 17 patients with *transversal* fractures, 16 had become completely deaf. The remaining patient showed some residual hearing. In 1 of the patients, the vestibular organ was calorically still excitable, but in 11 others, the vestibular function was completely abolished. In the 5 remaining patients, nothing was known in this regard, since vestibular tests could not be conducted immediately after the trauma, and patients did not report for the control examination either.

8 of the 122 ears with *longitudinal* fractures were completely deaf. In 2 of them, there was no remaining vestibular function either, but 3 others were calorically excitable, and in the remaining 3 there was no information about the outcome of the vestibular function tests. In 1 patient, the involved ear showed a sensorineural deafness; calorically, it could not be excited either. Hence, it was in only 9 patients with longitudinal fractures that either or both inner-ear functions were completely abolished (7%), whereas both functions were absent in *all* patients with transversal fractures (100%).

Cochlear function was graded in the following manner [99]: (a) normal hearing; (b) high-tone loss or a 4-kHz notch of at least 40 dB (*Escher*'s type II); (c) flat hearing loss of at least 40 dB (*Escher*'s type III); (d) complete deafness.

According to table LVII, 42 patients of the present group with longitudinal fractures showed cochlear losses (35%). In an attempt to correlate the cochlear impairment with the severity of the original trauma, the injuries

Table LVI. Longitudinal and transversal temporal bone fractures: endocranial complications (percentages given in parentheses)

	Longitudinal fractures (n = 122)	Transversal fractures (n = 17)	All laterobasal fractures (n = 143)
Cerebrospinal fluid discharge from the ear Of these:	13 (11)	6 (35)	20 (14)
Fistula surgically closed	2 (2)	3 (18)	6 (4)
Otogenic meningitis	6 (5)	1 (6)	7 (5)

Table LVII. Cochlear function in 122 patients with longitudinal temporal bone fractures of various severity (percentages given in parentheses)

Cochlear function	Fracture without commotio cerebri	Fracture with commotio cerebri	Fracture with endocranial complications	Fracture, no details given
Normal (n = 75; 65)	5 (100)	25 (62.5)	12 (50)	33 (69)
High-frequency loss (Escher, type II) (n = 30; 25)	–	14 (35)	7 (29)	9 (19)
Flat loss (Escher, type III) (n = 4; 3)	–	–	3 (13)	1 (2)
Very profound loss (n = 8; 7)	–	1 (2.5)	2 (8)	5 (10)
Total (n = 117; 100)	5 (100)	40 (100)	24 (100)	48 (100)
Not known (n = 5)	–	2	2	1

were subdivided in longitudinal fractures *without* apparent endocranial complications (i.e. without concussions) and those *with* endocranial complications (except for FN palsies). Admittedly, this classification is rather gross; however, it permitted to group patients with sufficient accuracy, in spite of the large number of 49 patients, for whom no information was available. As is seen in table LVII, the percentage of patients with normal cochlear function decreased considerably with the increasing severity of the trauma. Hence, there was indeed a positive correlation. FN injuries also belong under the present heading. On account of their complexity, however, they will be discussed separately in chapter 5.4.4.

5.4.2. Roentgenological Findings

The X-ray findings were evaluated in blind study fashion, as was explained in chapter 2.3.2. In this manner, the clinical findings and the roentgenological ones were independently assessed. In many patients, for whom X-ray pictures had been made elsewhere and were therefore no longer available, new pictures were never taken. Hence, the figures cited in the present chapter differ in some instances considerably from those given in the previous chapters.

In 82 patients, the X-ray pictures of both mastoids in the Schüller projection were evaluated and, if available, those of both TB in the Stenvers projection. The results were written down and were later correlated with the physical findings demonstrated clinically and/or surgically. The criteria used for the assessment of *longitudinal* fractures were: an adequate trauma, a step in the posterosuperior wall of the external canal, marginal ruptures of the TM and, if present, an FN palsy. The criteria used for the assessment of *transversal* fractures were: an adequate trauma, a normal-appearing TM or a hemotympanum, loss of vestibular and cochlear functions and an FN paralysis. In both instances, the evidence was judged sufficient if in a given patient three of the four criteria were found to be valid.

Clinical diagnoses based on this method are not absolutely reliable as was demonstrated by 1 of the present cases. Following a traffic accident, a longitudinal TB fracture was diagnosed, the clinical evidence being a brain concussion, bleeding from the ear and an FN paralysis, while cochlear and vestibular functions were preserved. The Schüller X-ray picture did not reveal any fracture line. Neither could it be demonstrated during the course of the surgical decompression of the FN.

If one disregards the case just described, there were 67 longitudinal TB fractures that were diagnosed either clinically or surgically. It should be noted that 3 of the 35 fractures verified during surgery did not satisfy the above clinical criteria.

Table LVIII gives the assessment of the mastoid X-ray pictures after *Schüller*. As is shown in the table, one quarter of the longitudinal fractures were missed by the X-ray examination. However, there was no difference in this respect between the diagnosis made clinically and that made surgically, indicating that the clinical criteria were not really inferior to the surgical ones, in spite of the case just cited. In 1 patient, a fracture detected during surgery had been missed in the inspection of the Schüller X-ray picture. It was finally demonstrated in tomographic pictures subsequently taken.

Table LVIII. X-Ray findings in 67 patients with longitudinal temporal bone fractures (Schüller projection; percentages given in parentheses)

	Number of fractures	Positive X-ray findings	Negative X-ray findings
Total	67 (100)	50 (75)	17 (25)
Diagnosed clinically	32 (100)	24 (75)	8 (25)
Diagnosed surgically	35 (100)	26 (74)	9 (26)

Table LIX presents the evaluation of the *Stenvers* X-ray pictures in the 7 patients with transversal fractures. Although the total number is quite small, table LIX indicates that the roentgenological confirmation of transversal fractures is rather difficult. One fracture diagnosed clinically could not even be demonstrated by subsequent tomography.

The reverse situation, i.e. that a *longitudinal* fracture was diagnosed by X-rays, but that corresponding clinical signs and symptoms were absent, was encountered 4 times. In none of these patients, however, were there any reasons for a surgical exploration that might have provided final verification. *Transversal* fractures were diagnosed by X-rays in 3 cases, in which there were no corresponding clinical signs or symptoms. In 1 of these 3, the fracture was not verified surgically either (table LX).

These findings may be summarized by stating that the roentgenological confirmation of *longitudinal* TB fractures by means of mastoid X-rays was positive in 75%; false-positive results were obtained in 7%. In only 57% of the *transversal* fractures, however, a positive confirmation was made, and the percentage of false-positive results was as high as 43%.

Table LIX. X-Ray findings in 7 patients with transversal temporal bone fractures (Stenvers projection; percentages given in parentheses)

	Number of fractures	Positive X-ray findings	Negative X-ray findings
Total	7 (100)	4 (57)	3 (43)
Diagnosed clinically	5 (100)	2 (40)	3 (60)
Diagnosed surgically	2 (100)	2 (100)	–

Table LX. Temporal bone fractures diagnosed by X-rays: correlation with clinical and surgical findings (percentages given in parentheses)

	Longitudinal fracture	Transversal fracture
Diagnosed by X-rays	55 (100)	7 (100)
Confirmed clinically or surgically	51 (93)	4 (57)
Clinically not confirmed	4 (7)	2 (29)
Surgically not confirmed	–	1 (14)
Not confirmed, total	4 (7)	3 (43)

5.4.3. Endocranial Complications

As was already mentioned, discharge of blood toward the outside invariably ceased on its own in all of our patients and did not require any special therapeutic measures. In 2 patients, however, endocranial hemorrhages had developed that required surgery. In 1 case, a subdural hematoma was found, accompanied by an FN paralysis, and in the other an epidural hematoma, which extended into the cranial vault. Both had occurred after longitudinal fractures and were drained by neurosurgical approaches.

In 31 patients with laterobasal skull fractures, the dura was lacerated. In 1 case, the dura had remained intact, but it had prolapsed through a gap in the tegmen tympani. Discharge of CSF was observed in 14 patients — 11 with longitudinal fractures and 3 with transversal fractures. It ceased spontaneously, generally around the end of the first week, except in 1 case, in which it did not stop until after the fourth month. (Since no surgery was performed, no statement about the site of the underlying lesion can be made.) 6 fistulae were surgically exposed and closed by means of free muscle transplants. 2 of them were located in the region of the tegmen tympani and a third over the roof of an old mastoidectomy cavity. All 3 were associated with longitudinal fractures. In the remaining 3 cases, the labyrinth was split by a lateral transversal fracture and the CSF entered the middle ear via this fracture. 1 of these labyrinthine fistulae had not closed itself on its own 7 months after the trauma.

In 7 patients, an otogenic meningitis was brought about by an infection ascending via a dura gap. Interestingly enough, in none of these cases had the meningitis been preceded by discharge of CSF from the ear. In 6 patients, the dura defect had been produced by a *longitudinal* fracture — in 3 of them, the fracture was extensive, accompanied by considerable soft-tissue lacerations and signs of brain injury. In 1 case, necrotic brain tissue had prolapsed into the ME via a fracture in the tegmen tympani and a tear in the dura. 5 of these meningitis cases developed during the first 9 days after the trauma, 1 each on the third, fifth or seventh days and 2 on the ninth day. All 5 were successfully treated by surgical debridement of the ME and mastoid, closure of the defect and antibiotic therapy. The sixth case developed after a symptom-free interval of 16 years, following an earlier longitudinal fracture. The port of entry was a dura defect in the region of the antrum. In the seventh case, it developed on the second day after a lateral *transversal* fracture. The infectious material had entered via the fractured labyrinth. The meningitis cleared up after the fracture was covered by muscle and fascia transplants.

In 1 patient with a longitudinal fracture, a dura tear was detected during surgery right above the tegmen of the antrum. It was virtually obstructed by necrotic brain tissue, which had prolapsed into the ME. There was no discharge of CSF. The necrotic tissue was sucked away and the defect closed with lyophilized dura and a muscle transplant. The same method was employed in the case already mentioned with meningitis and a brain-tissue prolapse into the ME. Healing was uneventful in both cases and no functional cerebral impairments remained.

In another patient with a longitudinal fracture, but without discharge of CSF, an intradural pneumatocele was demonstrated roentgenologically. The same trauma had also caused an FN paralysis. During surgery, the nerve was found crushed in the vicinity of the geniculate ganglion. It was decompressed and the dura gap, located in the same region, was closed.

In one further patient, an extradural pneumatocele was discovered, 35 years after a gunshot injury, involving the temporal bone. It had rendered the ear completely deaf and paralyzed the FN. The old X-ray pictures clearly demonstrated that the pneumatocele had developed *after* this long time interval. During surgery, it was found that the bullet had penetrated the Fallopian canal and the sigmoid sinus and had separated the mastoid tip from its body. The sigmoid sinus, which did no longer carry any blood, had apparently established a connection between the extradural space and the mastoid air cells and, in this manner, had led to the development of the pneumatocele. The communication could be successfully closed by a muscle transplant.

1 patient with a brain abscess that had developed after a laterobasal skull fracture was lost to follow-up. A brain infarction of traumatic origin was diagnosed once, following a longitudinal temporal bone fracture. There was no death in this group of patients with endocranial complications. Table LXI presents a summary of all endocranial complications described in the foregoing.

5.4.4. Facial Nerve Lesions

With the exception of 1 patient, who suffered from a facial tic 5 years after a longitudinal TB fracture, all the 100 traumatic FN lesions seen manifested themselves as paralyses. In most of them, the function recovered completely, either spontaneously or after surgical intervention. In 5 patients, a circumscribed lesion of the nerve could be demonstrated. In 1 case already mentioned, the nerve, apparently lying free in an old mastoidectomy cavity, was injured in the region of the second knee. Surgical exploration revealed

Table LXI. Endocranial complications in 143 patients with laterobasal skull fractures

Dura prolapse	1		
CSF discharge from ear, fistula spontaneously closed	14 ⎫	20	(14%)
CSF discharge from ear, fistula surgically closed	6 ⎭		
Meningitis	6		
Meningitis and brain prolapse	1		
Brain prolapse	1		
Pneumatocele	1		
Total number of dura defects	30		(21%)
Extradural pneumatocele	1		
Temporal lobe infarction	1		
Endocranial hemorrhage	2		
Total number of endocranial complications	34		(24%)

that only a small number of the nerve fibers was actually severed. Function returned completely to normal within a year.

In 3 patients, gunshot injuries of the mastoid, that had occurred 30 years earlier, had produced dead ears and severed the nerve in its mastoid portion. These ears were operated on for various other reasons (e.g. cholesteatoma, extradural pneumatocele). Reconstruction of the nerves was not attempted.

A nerve injury occurred via the transtympanal route, when a child fell onto a pair of scissors that entered the EEC. The labyrinth was destroyed, rendering the ear deaf. The FN had been severed in its tympanal portion. 1 year after the surgical repair and the rerouting of the nerve, the resting tonus was symmetrical on both sides, but the facial mobility on the side of the injury was still less that on the other.

FN palsies had developed in 95 patients, following blunt head trauma. In 6 of them, a TB fracture, although suspected, could not be verified either clinically or roentgenologically. Since the function recovered spontaneously, surgical exploration was not carried out so that the place of the suspected lesion was never established. In 3 more cases, the nerve was decompressed surgically, but the place of the injury was not demonstrated (recovery after 3 weeks in 1 case; in the 2 others, the outcome was not known).

In the 86 palsies that remain, identification of the fracture was facilitated either by the clinical and roentgenological findings (17 longitudinal fractures and 5 transversal ones) or the paralysis could be correlated with a certain type of fracture during surgery. Longitudinal fractures had caused 67 of them, transversal fractures 15 and mastoid fractures 4 (table LXII). This means that 55% of the 122 longitudinal fractures observed were accompanied by an FN palsy and so were 88% of the transversal fractures. Two patients had suffered bilateral pareses; in 1 of them, bilateral longitudinal fractures were demonstrated surgically.

In 3 patients with longitudinal fractures and FN palsies that were explored surgically, a luxated incus was found that was compressing the FN in its tympanal portion. In 1 case, the fracture had run twice across the nerve canal, i.e. in the region of the geniculate ganglion as well as in the mastoid portion. In 9 patients with longitudinal fractures and in 1 with a transversal one, the place of injury of the nerve could not be detected. The

Table LXII. Facial nerve paralysis in 100 patients: mode of injury

Mode of injury	Diagnosis established	Number of patients
Longitudinal temporal bone fracture	surgically	50
	clinically/roentgenologically	17
Transversal fracture	surgically	10
	clinically/roentgenologically	5
Mastoid fracture	surgically	4
No fracture	surgically	3
	clinically/roentgenologically	6
Gunshot injury	surgically	3
Transtympanal injury	surgically	1
Iatrogenic injury (cleaning of mastoid cavity)	surgically	1

Table LXIII. Facial nerve injuries: location confirmed during surgery (percentages given in parentheses)

Type of temporal bone fracture	Geniculate ganglion	Tympanal portion	2nd knee	Mastoid portion
Longitudinal (n = 39)	31 (80)	2 (5)	4 (10)	2 (5)
Transversal (n = 9)	4 (45)	2 (22)	3 (33)	–
Total (n = 48)	35 (73)	4 (8)	7 (15)	2 (4)

types of lesion established in the remaining 48 cases are listed in table LXIII.

With longitudinal fractures and medial transversal fractures, the place of predilection for FN lesions was definitely the region of the geniculate ganglion. Lateral transversal fractures injured the nerve at the place where they traversed the medial wall of the tympanic cavity, i.e. at the border between the vestibular and cochlear portions of the labyrinth — or, with respect to the nerve, in its tympanal portion above the oval window or in the region of the second knee.

In 33 cases, the *time of onset* of the paralysis could not be determined any more for the reasons repeatedly mentioned. When patients were unconscious at admittance, voluntary nerve action could of course not be tested. In some other patients, soft-tissue swellings probably prevented the examiner to notice a loss of FN function. The times of onset of the remaining 62 pareses were ordered in the following groups, according to the scheme proposed by *von Schulthess* [378]: *immediate* onset (on the day of the accident), *early* onset (within the first 3 days) and *late* onset (after the third day). The distribution for the various types of lesions under discussion is listed in table LXIV. According to table LXIV, late onsets prevailed with longitudinal fractures (51%) and immediate onsets with transversal fractures (57%). However,

Table LXIV. Facial nerve paralysis: time of onset for various types of causes (percentages given in parentheses)

Time of onset	Longitudinal fractures (n = 67)		Transversal fractures (n = 15)	Mastoid fractures (n = 4)	Type of fracture not clearly established (n = 9)
	direct (n = 64)	incus luxation (n = 3)			
Immediate 21 (34)	14 (33)	–	4 (57)	1	2
Early 13 (21)	7 (16)	2	2 (29)	–	2
Late 28 (45)	22 (51)	1	1 (14)	1	3
Total 62 (100)	43 (100)	3	7 (100)	2	7
Unknown 33	21	–	8	2	2

this correlation did not constitute a unique sign for either form of fracture.

As was already mentioned, most traumatically induced FN injuries were explored surgically. The decision to perform surgery was made when percutaneous electrostimulation indicated a definite loss of excitability or when the ear in question had to be operated on for some other reason. According to the method recommended by *Wullstein* [471], a simple mastoidectomy was usually performed first. Thereafter, a search was made for the fracture line. When found, it was followed up to the point where it crossed the Fallopian canal. This region was debrided, the nerve exposed and its sheath slit open. In the same session, a CSF fistula, if present, was closed, and the ossicular chain reconstructed. Occasionally, the epitympanum had to be opened from a transmeatal approach in order to assure access to the geniculate ganglion. In 1 case, the transtemporal route was the only possible way to the ganglion.

If the place of injury could not be demonstrated, the nerve was invariably exposed widely between the geniculate ganglion and the second knee and to some extent also in its mastoid portion. To slit the nerve sheath open appeared to be a logical step, not only because the nerve might become edematous after surgery, but also because in 1 patient a discontinuity, 1 cm in length, was uncovered in this manner. The gap was completely filled with blood coagula. Without opening the nerve sheath, it would not have been detected. In this particular case, the gap was bridged by interposing an autologous transplant taken from the major auricular nerve. In 2 other patients, in whom an FN discontinuity was found, the nerve was rerouted, since both ears were completely deaf. One lesion had been caused by a lateral transversal fracture and the other by a transmeatal injury.

In 2 patients, an old longitudinal fracture of long standing was accidentally detected during the course of ME reconstruction for the improvement of hearing. Both fractures had involved the geniculate ganglion. Since FN pareses had also existed for many years (12 or 30 years, respectively), nerve decompression was not attempted.

If one examines the functional postsurgical results in relation to the type of fracture found (leaving out the 2 cases just described), one must conclude that the prognosis is much more favorable with longitudinal fractures than with transversal ones (table LXV).

In table LXV, a *good* result meant that the resting tonus was bilaterally equal and that the active mobility of the facial musculature was also equal on the two sides, or nearly so; a *moderate* result that a distinct difference existed between the two sides with respect to their active mobility; and a *poor* result when even the resting tonus was unequal on the two sides.

The functional results after nerve repair were correlated with the site of the nerve injury (table LXVI). However, this relation did not yield any prognostic clues. (The case in which the nerve was injured in two separate places was omitted from table LXVI. After 2 years, function had returned to a moderate degree.)

In addition to the results of electrical stimulation, the *time of onset* is usually considered an important prognostic sign, i.e. the earlier the onset, the worse the prognosis. In the present series, the functional results were clearly inferior for pareses of immediate onset as compared to those of early or late

Table LXV. Functional results of facial nerve surgery in 70 patients with longitudinal and transversal temporal bone fractures (percentages given in parentheses)

	Results			
	good	moderate	poor	unknown
Longitudinal fractures (n = 65)	27 (54)	20 (40)	3 (6)	15
Transversal fractures (n = 15)	3 (25)	7 (58)	2 (17)	3

Table LXVI. Functional results of facial nerve surgery for various sites of injury (percentages given in parentheses)

Location	Results			
	good	moderate	poor	unknown
Geniculate ganglion (n = 32)	13 (59)	9 (41)	–	10
Tympanal portion (n = 8)	3 (60)	1 (20)	1 (20)	3
2nd knee (n = 70)	3 (50)	2 (33)	1 (17)	1
Mastoid portion (n = 5)	3 (60)	2 (40)	–	–
Unknown (n = 41)	22 (67)	10 (30)	1 (3)	8
Total (n = 93)	44 (62)	24 (34)	3 (4)	22

onset, but even in the latter two groups good recovery occurred in only 60% of all cases (table LXVII).

A comparison of the results achieved in the surgically treated group with those obtained in the nonsurgically treated group (in which the FN palsy was left to recover spontaneously) is of course not capable of demonstrating the superiority of one or the other method. The surgically treated group included cases in which the nerve could no longer be excited, i.e. cases with an a priori poor prognosis, whereas in all cases not submitted to surgery excitability was preserved and the prognosis was therefore judged to be favorable. However, there was a testable proposition, i.e. whether or not, in retrospect, most cases with a poor prognosis were indeed operated on, i.e. whether or not the indication for surgery was based on correct criteria. As demonstrated in table LXVIII, good functional recovery occurred more often (i.e. by about

Table LXVII. Functional results of facial nerve surgery: role of the time on onset of the paralysis (percentages given in parentheses)

Time of onset	Results			
	good	moderate	poor	unknown
Immediate (n = 22)	8 (42)	9 (47)	2 (11)	3
Early (n = 13)	6 (60)	4 (40)	–	3
Late (n = 28)	12 (63)	7 (37)	–	9
Unknown (n = 30)	12 (48)	10 (40)	3 (12)	5
Total (n = 93)	38 (52)	30 (41)	5 (7)	20

Table LXVIII. Facial nerve paralysis: comparison of functional results of surgical and nonsurgical measures (percentages given in parentheses)

Management	Results			
	good	moderate	poor	unknown
Surgical (n = 65)	22 (46)	21 (45)	4 (9)	18
Nonsurgical (n = 28)	16 (61)	9 (35)	1 (4)	2
Total (n = 93)	38 (52)	30 (41)	5 (7)	20

one quarter) in the group left to recover spontaneously than in that submitted to surgery. Admittedly, however, even in the first group the functional results were still poor in about one third of the cases.

The functional results were not only determined by the fact whether or not the nerve was surgically decompressed or by the question if the indication for surgery was correctly made. They were also affected by the *time interval* between the trauma and the surgical intervention (table LXIX).

The first week after the trauma was taken as the earliest interval, since only 3 patients were operated within the first 3 days. Although the numbers are too small for a reliable statistical evaluation, table LXIX suggests that the results of early decompression might be considerably better than average. During the second week already, the chances for recovery appeared to decrease, to become definitely worse after the 3-month limit. It should be pointed out especially that the results of early decompression (73% good results) appeared to be even better than those obtained by conservative management (61% good results; cf. also table LXVIII).

One general problem with post facto clinical assessments lies in the considerable variation in the time of postsurgical observations. *Krekorian* [256], who limited himself exclusively to nerve suture and autotransplantation, asserted that final results could only be assessed after a postsurgical interval of at least 16 months.

Of our group of 93 patients, 20 did not present themselves for the con-

Table LXIX. Facial nerve surgery: correlation between functional results and time of surgery after the injury (percentages given in parentheses)

	Results			
	good	moderate	poor	unknown
0–1 week (n = 17)	8 (73)	3 (27)	–	6
1–3 weeks (n = 22)	6 (35)	9 (53)	2 (12)	5
3 weeks to 3 months (n = 23)	7 (44)	8 (50)	1 (6)	7
> 3 months (n = 4)	1 (25)	1 (25)	2 (50)	–
Total (n = 65)	22 (46)	21 (45)	4 (9)	18

trol examination, as is evident from the preceding tables. Of the remaining 73, several had their final evaluation already within a few weeks after surgery. Others remained under clinical observation for a year or more on an outpatient basis. After axonomatmesis, one cannot expect reinnervation before 3–6 months [115, 299]. It must therefore be assumed that for some of the results labeled moderate or poor in the foregoing tables the time of observation was too brief, not permitting a final assessment.

For these reasons, the results, as listed in table LXX, are ordered according to the time of the final examination. As may be seen, the duration of postsurgical observation was 3 months or shorter in about 45% of all patients. However, the results obtained were not markedly different from those found after the longer period of between 3 months and 1 year. After the first year, however, the results became decidely poorer. The explanation for these startling findings cannot lie in the fact that good functional results, obtained earlier, deteriorated later. The only logical interpretation appears to be that the majority of patients, provided they presented themselves at all for a control examination, continued to come in until either of two conditions were fulfilled: (a) that they themselves were satisfied with the functional result or (b) that physician and patient were convinced that further improvements could no longer be expected. This assumption would explain why, on the average, patients with poor functional results required longer periods of postsurgical observation than those with good results. These considerations permit one to conclude that, at least in a large portion of the patients that were reexamined at all, the last result listed in their record reflects the final state of recovery fairly well and that the analyses, as presented in the foregoing, are sufficiently valid.

Table LXX. Facial nerve paralysis: functional results — duration of postsurgical observation (percentages given in parentheses)

	Results		
	good	moderate	poor
Up to 3 weeks (n = 8)	5 (62)	3 (38)	–
3 weeks to 3 months (n = 25)	13 (52)	11 (44)	1 (4)
3 months to 1 year (n = 20)	14 (70)	5 (25)	1 (5)
> 1 year (n = 21)	6 (29)	11 (57)	3 (14)
Total (n = 73)	38 (52)	30 (41)	5 (7)

5.5. Postmortem Findings

As may be recalled from chapter 2.2, 89 TB specimens were examined with special emphasis on the effects of skull trauma. 23 *TB fractures* were found; 18 of them longitudinal, 2 transversal and 3 atypical in direction. *Fissures* in the medial tympanic wall were seen in 3 cases.

All of the 18 *longitudinal fractures* ran across the roof of the antrum. 2 of them continued toward the *posterior* rim of the petrous pyramid; the remaining 16, however, continued in an *anteromedial* direction, shifting their course above the tubal ostium, to follow along the *anterior* rim of the petrous pyramid in a medial direction. Hence, within the petrous portion, the *general* course of the fractures was fairly uniform. However, there was quite some variation in the tympanic portion.

In 5 of the cases, the longitudinal fracture did neither involve the EEC nor the tympanic annulus, its most lateral end point being somewhere in the tegmen typani or in the mastoid. In 5 other cases, the roof of the EEC was completely torn off, separating Shrapnell's membrane from the remainder of the TM (cf. chapter 3.4.4). In only 8 cases did a fracture line exist in the posterosuperior wall of the EEC, running parallel to its axis. 3 of these latter fractures were covered by intact skin. In 3 others, the skin was torn along the fracture line, but the TM was intact. In only 2 cases did the soft-tissue defect continue onto the posterosuperior quadrant of the TM. If one would assume for the moment that the patients with the torn-off roof of the external canal could have survived — which is not very probable, considering the severity of the trauma — a step in the posterior wall of the EEC would have been observed clinically in a maximum of 13 cases. (Since in 3 of them no dislocation was present, probably no step would have become tangible.)

Hemorrhages from the involved ear had occurred in 10 cases. In 10 of the 11 cases with intact TM, there was a hemotympanum. Hemotympana were also found associated with: lateral transversal fractures; fissures of the medial tympanic wall; fractures in the immediate neighborhood (lateral cranial vault or skull basis); and also, in 1 case, with a contralateral longitudinal TB fracture and with 10 blunt skull injuries, which had not directly involved the ME or its immediate environment. Finally, there were 3 TM ruptures associated with blunt skull traumata that had not produced any TB fractures (cf. chapter 3.4.4). These findings indicate that hemotympana and hemorrhages from the ear are important, but by no means invariable, clues for the presence of fractures in the region of the otobasis (table LXXI).

The two *transversal* fractures included a lateral fracture and a medial one. The *lateral* fracture had split the labyrinth, the fracture line running across both cochlear windows; the stapes footplate and the anterior crus were broken and the FN was severed above the oval window. There was a hemotympanum, but the TM was intact. The *medial* fracture ran through the fundus of the internal canal, splitting the cochlea open; the TM was likewise intact, but there was no hemotympanum. However, no statement about a peripheral FN injury can be made, since all nerves were torn in the inner meatus during the preparation.

2 of the 3 *atypical* fractures deserve special mention. 1 of them had been produced by a gunshot that had fractured the posterosuperior wall of the EEC lengthwise; the canal skin was torn and so was the adjacent part of the TM; however, the fracture line extended medially only as far as the tegmen tympani. The petrous bone was not involved at all. In the second case, the floor of the EEC was elevated by the fracture, the skin torn and there was a central TM rupture in the anteroinferior quadrant. The osseous tympanic annulus and the fibrocartilaginous annulus were both intact and there were no injuries in the ME.

In the third atypical fracture, the roof of an old radical mastoidectomy cavity was split open by a fracture running transversally to the longitudinal axis of the TB. (The structures within the ME had of course been removed during the previous operation.) The medial tympanic wall was well epithelialized and the labyrinth and the petrous portion were not injured. Among the total of 89 specimens, there was 1 more with an old mastoid cavity, but without a fracture.

1 of the 3 *fissures* involved the pyramidal process; the ME proper was

Table LXXI. Otological findings in 89 postmortem specimens after severe skull trauma

	Fracture of the external canal	13
Longitudinal temporal bone fractures (n = 18)	Soft tissue lacerations in the external canal	10
	Tympanic membrane rupture	7
	Hemotympanum	10
No TB fracture present (n = 71)	Fracture of external canal and soft tissue lacerations	2
	Tympanic membrane rupture	3
	Hemotympanum	15

undamaged. In the 2 other cases, they were located in the window region. In 1 of them, it ran from the rim of the RW for about 5 mm in a posterior direction; the ME was not involved. In the other, the fissure connected the inferior rim of the OW with the superior rim of the RW. A longitudinal TB fracture was also present.

What were the relations of the fracture lines to the FN? 1 of the fissures, as already mentioned, ran through the pyramidal process. In that particular case, the nerve could have been compressed by a hematoma, had the patient survived. With the fractures, longitudinal as well as transversal ones, the evidence is clearer: in the case of the lateral transversal fracture, the FN was torn in its tympanal portion. Whether or not the medial transversal fracture had produced a tangible nerve injury could not be established for the reasons already given. If the nerve was indeed injured, the injury should have occurred in the fundus of the internal meatus.

10 of the 18 longitudinal fractures did not involve the FN; 7 exposed the geniculate ganglion, apparently without grossly injuring the nerve. In all these cases, however, severe traction must have been exerted on the major superficial petrosal nerve, where it traversed the fracture line. There were some bone chips, and hematomata were visible directly on the ganglion. Therefore, some axons might have been severed. This notion is supported by the findings in the eighth case, in which the nerve was clearly injured. The fracture line crossed directly over the geniculate ganglion and there was a hematoma within the nerve sheath. Table LXXII summarizes the causes of the FN injuries, i.e. of those actually demonstrated and of those merely suspected.

Table LXXII. Causes of facial nerve injuries, demonstrated or suspected

Causes	
Transversal temporal bone fractures	2
Nerve torn in tympanal portion	1
Nerve damaged in internal meatus	(1) ?
Longitudinal temporal bone fractures	18
Nerve damaged in region of geniculate ganglion	8
Atypical fractures and fissures	6
Nerve damaged in mastoid portion	(1) ?

5.6. Discussion of Results

The clinical-surgical results as well as the postmortem findings fully confirm the conclusions drawn by the older, classical authors [190, 262, 442, 443, 452]: The majority of all *fractures* at the otobasis followed one of three typical routes: (a) along the anterior rim of the petrous pyramid (longitudinal fractures); (b) through the fundus of the internal meatus (medial transversal fracture), or (c) directly through the labyrinth between the vestibular and cochlear portions (lateral transversal fracture). The numerical ratio between longitudinal and transversal fractures was similar to that given in the literature: 88:12 for the clinical cases and 90:10 for the postmortem specimens.

Among the atypical forms, mastoid fractures were found in 4 of the clinical patients. (This type was specially mentioned by *Voss* [450].) Furthermore, there was 1 clinical patient and 1 postmortem specimen, each with a compressed fracture of the floor of the EEC; and, once more in a clinical patient and also in a postmortem specimen, there was a fracture of the roof of an old mastoid cavity. Such a cavity apparently constitutes a (nonphysiological) locus minoris resistentiae.

Fissures in the region of the RW were found in 1 patient during surgery and in 2 postmortem specimens. Apparently, when the lateral skull basis receives a blunt trauma, the labyrinthine capsule is subjected to strong bending stresses.

Brain concussion is numerically the most frequent sign of TB fractures. It was present in 94% of all cases. However, hemorrhages from the ear, steps in the osseous wall of the EEC and marginal TM ruptures are not infallible signs of longitudinal fractures. In a considerable number of fractures that were demonstrated either during surgery or in the postmortem examinations, they were not present. On the other hand, hemorrhages and TM ruptures were occasionally found, either separately or in combination, in the *absence* of longitudinal fractures.

The loss of one or both *inner-ear functions* appears to be quite a reliable sign for the existence of a transversal fracture. It remains to be seen, however, whether the inner-ear functions may also be preserved, even if such fractures are present. (In that case, the fractures would probably not be recognized as such.) Furthermore, the X-ray findings are not absolutely reliable with respect to the demonstration of transversal fractures. And only lateral fractures are always accompanied by hematomata, which are much less frequent with medial fractures. Postmortem examinations indicated that hemotympana may be produced by a variety of different injuries to the lateral skull region, which do not necessarily involve the ME and the TB.

In our cases, vestibulocochlear lesions could be demonstrated in all proven instances of transversal fractures. They were only found in 35% of the longitudinal fractures. In only 7% of the latter fractures, either or both functions were completely abolished. If they were partially preserved, the degree of impairment depended on the severity of the preceding trauma. In most cases, the impairment was rather slight.

In view of the observations reported by others, it was not surprising to learn that the *X-ray examination* had missed 25% of the longitudinal fractures and 47% of the transversal ones. Only *Boenninghaus* [39] and *Rohrt* [361] were able to achieve better results, i.e. 80 and 88% correct results, respectively. All other authors gave numbers lower than, or equal to, our own. It has been claimed [135, 317] that tomography provides better information about the existence of fractures, but in many cases it is questionable if the extra effort and the increased X-ray dosis are warranted, since even tomography is frequently incapable of exactly localizing an FN lesion or a dura fistula.

Discharge of CSF from the involved ear had occurred in 14% of the laterobasal fractures. This percentage is about equal to that given by *Escher* [102] for a group of 39 patients. All other authors reported considerably smaller percentages, with the exception of *Piquet* [345] and of *Roche* [360]. Significantly enough, there was no recognizable discharge from the ears in the 7 patients, who later developed a meningitis, although a dura defect could be demonstrated during surgery, and no discharge either in the patient with the intradural pneumatocele. It is highly probable therefore that in a number of additional cases clinically latent dura lesions were present, but were never identified.

The finding that the discharge of CSF from the ear ceased spontaneously in most cases, as a rule after about 1 week, also agrees with the experience of others, and so does the observation that, when the labyrinth was widely split open by a lateral transversal fracture, the fluid discharge either did not cease spontaneously at all, or only after a relatively long time interval.

The reported incidence of otogenic *meningitis*, 5% after laterobasal fractures, agrees with the percentage given by *Grete* [149] for 486 temporal bone fractures, but both percentages are low when compared to others cited in the literature. It ought to be noted that meningitis occurred in our patients with equal frequency after longitudinal as well as after transversal fractures, although transversal fractures are traditionally considered more dangerous in this respect. 6 of the 7 cases of meningitis developed early after the injury, i.e. between the second and ninth days. In 4 cases, the TB was virtually shattered; there were extensive soft-tissue lacerations and, in a fifth case, a prolapse of necrotic brain tissue as well. One might still debate therefore if preventive surgery, for the reconstruction of the pneumatized ME spaces, should not be carried out in every patient with such extensive injuries of the otobasis, as was originally recommended by *Voss* [450]. On the other hand, early surgery would subject these gravely injured patients, all of whom must have suffered severe brain traumata, to additional risks. In every case, therefore, the decision to perform surgery must be made on an individual basis.

The 2 patients reported — 1 in whom an otogenic meningitis developed 16 years after a longitudinal TB fracture, and the other in whom a pneumatocele appeared 35 years after a gunshot injury — should be of more than passing interest. The longest interval between a *longitudinal* fracture and a subsequent meningitis cited in the literature [127] is 1 year, although there are some reports about late ascending infections after *transversal* fractures [46, 372]. Extradural pneumatoceles of otogenic origin are quite rare. As far as we are aware, a late occurrence, as in our patient, has never been described.

In our present material, the incidence of *FN palsies*, in conjunction with longitudinal fractures (55%) as well as with transversal ones (88%), was quite high. Inspection of table LIV shows that the *ratio* between the two numbers (about 2:3) was approximately the same as that generally reported in the literature. In *absolute numbers*, however, both incidences were far higher than those reported elsewhere. This could have something to do with the fact that members of our department pay special attention to the existence of FN palsies (i.e. perhaps more than some others) because of their interest in surgical decompression. Another possibility might be that a relatively large number of patients with FN paralyses are being referred to our department, whereas those with uncomplicated fractures remain in primary- or secondary-care hospitals. The fact that in our postmortem material 8 longitudinal fractures, out of a total of 18 (44%), were accompanied by FN lesions, argues against the second of the above alternatives. On the other hand, the latter cases constituted a group with severe, and eventually lethal, injuries. Hence, the above question cannot be resolved. Be that as it may, the frequent association of FN palsies with longitudinal TB fractures persuaded us to consider it an important sign in the clinical diagnosis of such fractures (cf. chapter 5.4.2).

A survey of the clinical cases as well as of the postmortem specimens indicates that most of the FN injuries associated with *longitudinal* fractures took place in the region of the geniculate ganglion, i.e. 80% among the surgical cases and 100% in the postmortem specimens. This confirms the results of earlier postmortem findings [443] as well as surgical-clinical observations [79, 113, 189].

In the presence of *transversal* fractures, however, the region of the ganglion was only involved in about one half of all cases, since it is only the lateral fractures that are capable of injuring the nerve at the point where it emerges from the labyrinth, i.e. in its tympanal portion or in the region of the second knee. It is this region that is generally considered the place of predilection of *all* traumatic FN injuries [380].

In our experience, the FN was most frequently injured in the region of the geniculate ganglion. However, our percentage figures are smaller than those of *Fisch* [113], who found the ganglion involved in 93% of longitudinal fractures and in 90% of transversal fractures, and those of *Müller and Edel* [317], who found such involvement in 93 and 70%, respectively.

The difficulties one encounters when trying to determine the *site* of an FN injury from inspection of X-ray pictures were already mentioned. Therefore, it does not appear warranted to expose the geniculate ganglion immediately from a transtemporal approach as has been recommended [114, 388]. To start out by first performing a mastoidectomy, in an effort to find and then follow the fracture line, appears to be the best way to guide the surgeon to the place of the FN lesion which, in a fair number of cases, may be quite remote from the ganglion. If one does not detect the fracture line as it crosses the Fallopian canal, it is often helpful to expose the nerve widely in its tympanal and mastoid portions. The fissure at the pyramidal process found in 1 of our postmortem specimens suggests that a hematoma or an edema may occasionally occur in this region. There are added advantages in the transmastoid approach: it facilitates debridement of the mastoid and of the ME, if necessary; it may also be performed under local anesthesia, whereas the transtemporal approach requires general anesthesia.

Table LXVII had indicated that the prognosis of an immediate paresis is considerably worse than that of early and late pareses. *Fisch* [114] may be overstating his case when he says that this classification is obsolete. However, one must agree with his further statement, i.e. that the decision whether to decompress the nerve surgically or to manage a paresis conservatively should under no circumstances be based on the time of the first appearance of the paresis, but only on the results of the electrophysiological tests. Nevertheless, early decompression, i.e. within the first week, gave better results in our hands (73% good results) than waiting for spontaneous recovery, relying on the results of electrophysiological tests which had been favorable (61% good results). The good results of early surgery, together with the fact that results became worse in the second week, should persuade everyone, when being in doubt, to perform surgical decompressions early.

After late decompression, i.e. beyond the 3-month limit, good results were only obtained in individual patients. This has also been the experience of others, e.g. *Krekorian* [256], who reported a good result following a nerve transplantation 8 months after the original injury. Therefore, when early surgery was foregone for whatever reasons, one should always try a late decompression, if the indication is present (i.e. if a persisting nerve compression is suspected); but one must properly explain to the patient that the chances for a favorable result are somewhat reduced.

6. Stenosis of the External Canal, Posttraumatic Cholesteatoma and Tubal Dysfunction

It appears logical to discuss these three entities under the same heading, but separate from the complications of laterobasal skull fractures, which were described in the last chapter. Although they are three distinctly different entities, their common link is that they may develop after TB fractures, but that they appear rather *late* after the injury. Furthermore, atresia of the EEC and tubal dysfunction may contribute to the development of an ME cholesteatoma. Numerically, they are relatively rare.

Passow [339] already described *stenoses* of the EEC. They were caused by cauterizations, scalding injuries, local soft tissue lacerations and by compression fractures of the socket of the jaw joint. He differentiated stenoses caused by contracted scars from those produced by apposition of new bone. He also pointed out the difficulties encountered in, and the relatively poor success of, the treatment of such stenoses. Finally, he mentioned that ME infections located behind them have a poor chance to heal.

Imhofer [209] separated stenoses caused by the contraction of scars from those following adhesions between adjacent skin areas. (He thought the latter type would mainly occur after fractures of the EEC walls.) *Imhofer* [209] also pointed out that such stenoses may aggravate existing ME infections or render them chronic. However, he maintained that this could not be due to the impairment of the self-cleaning of the EEC.

Weber [456] mentioned that a genuine cholesteatoma might form behind an atresia of the EEC and that it may break into the ME through the TM or into the mastoid through the posterior wall.

On the other hand, *Hörbst* [198] considered the layers of desquamated epithelium, which may accumulate in an EEC with impaired self-cleaning, and the destructively growing cholesteatoma two separate entities.

Schwarz [386] took up *Weber*'s concept again. He maintained that a mass of desquamated epithelium accumulating in the EEC ought to exert a pressure on the epithelium and its osseous walls. In this manner, the epithelial mass should be converted into a true cholesteatoma that shows inflammatory reactions and grows in a destructive manner.

This concept received support from a study on experimental animals conducted by *Steinbach* [413]. *Steinbach* demonstrated that an occlusion of the EEC may lead to the invasion of keratinizing epithelium into the subepithelial layers of the canal skin and thus, eventually, to the formation of a cholesteatoma.

Moritsch [311] considered scar formation in the EEC the most frequent cause of stenoses. He recommended to widen them by excising concentric rings of tissue; one should further attempt to convert the circular scars into longitudinal ones and to cover the epithelial defects by means of free skin grafts. When osseous stenoses are present one should thin them down by means of a bone drill. *Steinbach* [412] stated that in rare instances the tympanic bone, after an earlier injury, may even undergo fibrous dysplasia. This could lead to a recurrence of the stenosis or even to a complete atresia.

Johnson et al. [216] described a stenosis of the EEC that had been brought about when the capitulum of the jaw bone was pushed into the anterior EEC wall. When the patient chewed, the EEC walls collapsed, producing a fluctuating, conductive hearing impairment.

Wittmaack [466] was the first to describe a *cholesteatoma* that had developed in a well-pneumatized TB, following an injury caused by a shell fragment. *Grahe* [147] described a similar case: a patient, who died from complications of a retrolabyrinthine cholesteatoma, 12 years after a gunshot injury of the TB. *Grahe* assumed that the bullet had carried epithelial tissue deep into the wound and that this epithelium had become the source of the cholesteatoma.

Kelemen [229] conducted histological studies on the TB of persons who had died immediately after they had sustained grave skull injuries. He found cyst-like formations in the various layers of the TM, filled by an exudate. He also saw ruptured TM with their margins rolled up and lacerations of the canal skin and of the ME mucosa as well. These findings prompted him to suggest that the fresh wound margins might adhere to one another and eventually form epithelialized cysts; keratinizing lamellae might be sloughed off into these cysts. He furthermore thought that the margins of a torn TM might attach themselves to ME structures; such attachments might act as guides for the ingrowth of epithelium into the ME. He finally felt that, after spontaneous closure of the TM, retraction pockets might come into being, in which cholesteatomata could develop, aided by the accumulation of epithelial lamellae and inflammatory reactions.

Actually, these various forms of cholesteatoma had been described in all details earlier by *Wittmaack* [466], and later once more by his student, *Steurer* [418], on the basis of their own histological studies.

In further pursuing the problem of the cholesteatoma development following mastoid injuries caused by bullets and shell fragments, *Weber* [456] raised the question why epithelial scattering and subsequent cholesteatoma formation did not seem to occur after *longitudinal* fractures. A year later, *Steurer* [418] described 2 relevant cases: posttraumatic cholesteatomata had developed after the destruction of the posterior EEC walls. 1 was detected 17 years after a bullet had passed through the canal wall, the other 9 years after a longitudinal fracture had left a cleft in the posterosuperior portion of the tympanic annulus. *Thulin* [432b] and *Nilsson* [329] each reported a similar case. Both of these cholesteatomata were detected 10 years after the original trauma.

2 other posttraumatic cholesteatomata of similar origin were described by *Escher* [99]. 1 had developed in the region of an old trephine opening in the squama made 20 years earlier; it had destroyed the posterior wall of the EEC. The other evolved from a longitudinal fracture. 16 years later, keratinizing epithelium was found to have invaded a cleft in the roof of the EEC. Although, in the second case, the cholesteatoma had clearly originated from the fracture, it had not followed the cleft in its further development, but had grown medially in the direction of the labyrinth partly destroying it in the process. Hence, this cholesteatoma, although of traumatic origin, had shown a growth tendency of its own.

A number of additional cholesteatomata were reported; all of them had originated from *longitudinal* fractures (1 case after 2 years [223]; 1 case after 3 years [392]; 2 cases after 3 or 4 years [376a]).

Eckel [89] described 4 cases of posttraumatic cholesteatoma. 2 of them had developed after bullets or shell fragments had become embedded in the mastoid, another after a longitudinal fracture of the TB, 13 years earlier, and the last after epithelial invasion, which had started from the margins of a TM perforation, originally produced by an air pressure insult. On the basis of his own findings and partly on *Kelemen*'s [229] old notions of 1934, he differentiated three modes of origin of traumatic cholesteatomata: (1) from epithelial scattering produced by a trauma (e.g. gunshot injury); (2) from epithelium that was hemmed-in within a fracture cleft, and (3) from epithelial migration (e.g. from an old TM rupture). A case report by *Strupler* [422] (cited by *Eckel* [90]) prompted him to add a fourth category: (4) from transplanted epithelium (e.g. when keratinizing epithelium had been transplanted into the ME mucosa, following a mechanical rupture of the TM that had subsequently healed over). *Eckel* was able to collect from the literature 17 other cholesteatomata that had originated from longitudinal TB fractures; their development took 1–24 years, an average of 9 years. The incidence of cholesteatoma thus generated was estimated to be 1 in 263 TB fractures, or 3 in 1,000 cholestatomata [381].

Escher [99] pointed out that in some rare cases pieces of TM epithelium might be scattered into the ME mucosa by the trauma, an accident that could also lead to the development of a cholesteatoma. *Wodak* [469] and *Schwarz* [386] thought this could only be possible when an inflammation would simultaneously exist in the ME. (*Wodak* developed this notion after following up on a TM injury that had originally been produced by a match-stick.) *Seaman and Newell* [390] saw 13 patients in whom keratinizing epithelium had been embedded in the ME mucosa following TM ruptures that were caused by air pressure insults. The incidence was given as 12% of all TM ruptures authors had seen during the Vietnam war. In 1 patient, they removed five cholesteatoma pearls from the ME, several months after the injury. The pearls had no apparent connection with the TM. *Pahor* [335] observed an epidermoid cyst of the TM 1 year after it had been ruptured and subsequently healed.

There are only a few published reports about trauma to the *Eustachian tube*. Occasionally, foreign bodies were found lodged in the tubal lumen, e.g. grains of cereals [176] or ascaris worms [414, 451]. *Passow* [339] as well as *Imhofer* [209] pointed to the danger of injuring the tubal mucosa during catheterization, which may lead to a peritubal emphysema; they furthermore mentioned that a piece of a bougie might break off and be stuck in the tube. *Passow* [339] collected 4 cases from the literature with tubal injuries caused by bullets or knives. He stated that a posttraumatic tubal occlusion, if persisting, might lead to an ME effusion that resists therapy. *Von Schulthess* [379] reported on 2 patients with tubal dysfunction and subsequent ME effusion, following severe fractures of the facial bones. *Escher* [99] described a patient who had been impaled in the middle of his face. A tubal occlusion had ensued and a mucoid, jellylike effusion was found in the ME.

6.1. Our Clinical Results

Among our patients, there were 7 with stenoses of the EEC, 22 with cholesteatomata and 2 with tubal dysfunctions. Since all numbers are rather small, brief case histories will be presented, instead of summarizing tables.

6.1.1. Stenoses of the External Canal

The 7 cases of EEC stenoses are presented in inverse order of the duration of their existence:

(1) Fracture of the anterior canal wall; subtotal osseous stenosis corrected surgically after 3.5 months; distal to the stenosis: EEC filled with detritus, EEC walls and TM intact; good surgical result.

(2) Longitudinal TB fracture, involving the anterior canal wall; osseous atresia of the EEC, surgically corrected after 6 months: detritus distal to the atresia; central TM perforation; no keratinizing epithelium detected in the ME; tympanoplasty, type I; the EEC remained wide postsurgically, but the TM perforation reoccurred.

(3) Patient bitten by a dog; pinna torn off; subtotal stenosis of the external canal; surgical excision after 1 ycar; external canal tightly packed with detritus; canal walls and TM intact; good surgical results.

(4) Blunt skull trauma with longitudinal TB fracture; pinna torn and crushed; ear completely deaf; 4 years later, surgical excision of the (soft tissue) canal stenosis; EEC filled with detritus; TM attached to the medial tympanic wall, except for small free areas in the tubal and fenestral regions; dura prolaps through the tegmen tympani, covered by stratified epithelium; no surgical intervention in the ME; entrance to the EEC widened after excision of the scar tissues.

(5) Infraction of the floor of the EEC; subtotal soft tissue stenosis; fetid-smelling secretion; after 5 years, excision of scar tissue; EEC filled with detritus, walls and TM intact; postsurgical result good after additional bouginage.

(6) Blunt skull trauma; pinna torn off; ear completely deaf; stenosis (scar tissue) of the canal entrance; 20 years later, plastic reconstruction of the EEC; canal filled with detritus, walls intact, central TM perforation, no stratified epithelium in the ME; good surgical result.

(7) Ear region injured by shell fragments; prior surgery elsewhere; ear completely deaf; fetid secretion; osseous stenosis surgically corrected after 25 years: pus and detritus in the EEC; walls intact; central TM perforation; no stratified epithelium in the ME; good surgical results.

If one first limits consideration to cases 1–4, one recognizes a pattern: depending on the duration of the stenosis, the distal portion of the EEC is gradually filled up with lamellae of epidermis, until eventually, i.e. after about 4 years, the TM is pushed inward and parts of the tympanic cavity become lined with stratified epithelium. In cases 5–7, however, in which the stenosis existed for much longer periods, an epithelial invasion of the subepithelial tissues of the EEC or of the ME mucosa had failed to materialize.

What sets these 3 cases apart was a chronic secretory infection of the EEC (case 5) or the ME (cases 6 and 7). It is conceivable that the secretion and the bacterial decomposition of the detritus facilitated its discharge, through the narrow, but still patent, stenosis.

6.1.2. Posttraumatic Cholesteatomata

Only 8 of the 22 cholesteatomata of traumatic origin clearly developed from TB fractures. The remaining 14 evolved without any apparent relation to fractures that might, or might not, have occurred earlier. The latter cases will be described first.

(8) Longitudinal fracture 2 months earlier; central TM perforation; keratinizing epithelium grown from the margins of the perforation onto incus and stapes.

(9) Barotrauma 7 years earlier; 2 tympanoplasties without success; subtotal defect of the TM with migration of keratinizing epithelium onto the promontory.

(10) Longitudinal fracture 14 years earlier; central TM perforation; keratinizing epithelium grown from its margins onto incus and stapes.

(11) Gunshot injury of the ear 27 years earlier; ear completely deaf; central TM perforation with keratinizing epithelium grown onto the promontory.

(12) Ear injured by the explosion of an artillery shell 32 years earlier; central TM perforation and hazelnut-size cholesteatoma in the additus.

(13) Ear injured by an explosion 32 years earlier; central TM perforation; keratinizing epithelium grown from its margins onto incus and stapes.

(14) Longitudinal TB fracture 50 years earlier; discharge from the ear since that time; subtotal TM defect with epithelial migration onto the medial tympanic wall.

It is of course a question whether all the alterations described were already manifest cholesteatomata or whether some of them were still in preliminary stages. One factor common to cases 8–14 was an ingrowth of keratinizing epithelium from the margins of a posttraumatic central TM perforation into the ME — something that occasionally is also seen with central perforations of different origins. With the exception of case 8, this ingrowth was observed many years after the original trauma. One may assume that in case 8 an inverted part of the torn TM made early and direct contact with incus and stapes and adhered there. The incidence of such epithelial ingrowth was a mere 1.3% of a total of 531 TM ruptures, i.e. it was very small.

(15) Blunt skull trauma 3 years earlier; no evidence for a TB fracture; cholesteatoma pearl behind an intact TM attached to the incus; erosion of the long incudal crus.

(16) Blunt skull trauma 16 years earlier; cholesteatoma in the attic behind an intact TM.

In cases 15 and 16, the cholesteatoma existed behind an *intact* TM. It is suggested that it developed on the basis of epithelial scattering into the ME through a ruptured TM that, subsequently, had healed over.

(17) Injury caused by a welding spark 9 months earlier; central TM perforation; cholesteatoma pearl at the umbo.

(18) Blunt skull trauma 3 years earlier; no evidence for a TB fracture; retraction pocket in the posterosuperior quadrant of the TM.

(19) Ear injured by a metal fragment 14 years earlier; marginal TM perforation in the posterosuperior quadrant with attic cholesteatoma.

(20) Ear injured during an explosion 30 years earlier; TM attached to the promontory; keratinizing epithelium grown into the retrotympanal spaces.

(21) Ear injured during an explosion 35 years earlier; retraction pocket in the posterosuperior quadrant of the TM.

In cases 17–21, one may argue if the conditions seen were really caused by the preceding trauma. Nevertheless, it is conceivable that in case 17 an epithelial cyst had developed behind the TM, as had been previously described [229, 335]. In some of the remaining cases, retraction pockets in the TM could have been brought about by the trauma; such pockets have also been described [22]. After the cyst or the pockets were filled with detritus, cholesteatomata might have developed.

The 8 cholesteatomata described in the following developed in direct relation to TB fractures:

(22) Destruction of the posterosuperior wall of the EEC caused by a blunt skull trauma; ear completely deaf; after 19 years, a cholesteatoma was detected, it had spread from the EEC into the mastoid.

(23) Ear injured by shell fragments, completely deaf; stenosis at the entrance to the EEC; after 58 years, cholesteatoma in the mastoid and in the shattered remnants of the posterior wall of the EEC.

(24) Medial portion of the posterior canal wall torn off and pushed anteriorly; 2 years later, cholesteatoma behind the fragments in ME and antrum.

(25) Longitudinal fracture; FN decompression; 4 years later, cholesteatoma in the antrum, medial to the fracture line.

(26) Longitudinal fracture, distended cleft in the posterosuperior wall of the EEC; after 15 months, cholesteatoma in the cleft.

(27) Middle part of the posterior canal wall shattered by a fracture; 2 years later, a cholesteatoma was detected here that had spread into tympanic cavity and antrum.

(28) Longitudinal fracture in the posterosuperior wall of the EEC; FN palsy; surgical decompression; after 2 more years, cholesteatoma in the fracture cleft.

(29) Longitudinal fracture in the posterosuperior wall of the EEC; ear completely deaf; 8 years later, cholesteatoma in fracture cleft and antrum.

In cases 22–29, the topographical relation between the cholesteatoma and the fracture cleft was obvious. In case 22 a cholesteatoma, originating in the EEC, had spread into the shattered mastoid. In case 23, the questions cannot be decided: (a) whether the epithelium entered by way of the shattered posterior canal wall, as in case 22, (b) whether epithelium was thrown into the ME by the trauma, in the sense of *Grahe* [147], or (c) whether the stenosis of the EEC played a causative role. In cases 24 and 25, the cholesteatomata apparently took their origin from epithelium scattered into the tympanic cavity. In cases 25–29, however, it developed directly in the fracture cleft, but grew from there in the direction of the antrum, as has been previously described [97].

The incidence of cholesteatoma originating from a TB fracture was 7% among the total of 122 patients with such fractures, that of cholesteatoma developing directly in the fracture cleft 3%. Both figures are considerably higher than those previously reported by *Eckel* [90].

6.1.3. Posttraumatic Tubal Dysfunction

There were only 2 cases with tubal dysfunction of traumatic origin in our group of patients:

(30) In the first patient, the soft palate had been injured by a shell fragment. In spite of primary wound care, the palate had been indurated and subsequently contracted; there was rhinolalia aperta. After 25 years, mucoid effusion in the right ME; the left TM had formed adhesions with the promontory; there were conductive impairments of 25 dB on the right and 40 dB on the left. Patient could not actively ventilate his ME. A drainage tube in the right TM brought some transient relief.

(31) In the second patient, 16 years after a longitudinal TB fracture, the tympanic cavity was found to be completely epithelialized, without any aeration at all. A large cholesteatoma had developed in the ME, growing into the

well-pneumatized mastoid. During surgery, the tube was found to be obstructed. A large mastoid cavity was fashioned. The contralateral ear was normal.

In both patients, there was tubal dysfunction, on a structural basis in patient 31 and on a functional basis in patient 30. In patient 31, the tube of 1 ear was completely obstructed, probably brought on by an injury (that in turn had been caused by a longitudinal TB fracture), in a way similar to what was described by *von Schulthess* [379] and by *Escher* [99]. The adhesions of the remaining TM on the promontory had, in a surprisingly short time, led to epithelialization of the tympanic cavity and, subsequently, to an epi- and retrotympanal cholesteatoma. In patient 30, the effusion in the right ear had apparently served to maintain the ME space, preventing the extreme TM retraction found in the left ear. Why there was no effusion in that ear is difficult to say. Perhaps, there was some minimal tubal function remaining, still capable of draining the ME passively, but incapable of active ventilation.

6.2. Discussion of Results

In hardly 2 cases of the posttraumatic cholesteatomata reported in the foregoing chapter did the disease take the same course. The above listing of patient histories demonstrated that a large variety of different traumatic effects may trigger the same reaction, i.e. lead to the formation of a cholesteatoma.

All modes of origin mentioned in the literature were observed: for instance, the pressure exerted in the EEC by the accumulating lamellae of keratinizing epithelium may gradually depress the TM and, in the long run, lead to an active proliferation of epithelium within the ME (case 4); the same sequence of events may take place when the ME pressure is chronically decreased due to a tubal obstruction (case 31); or the inverted margins of a ruptured TM attaching themselves to ME structures may form a guide for the ingrowth of epithelium (case 8). Furthermore, it is quite conceivable that the epithelial migration (or metastasis) may not start until many years after the trauma, as is suggested by cases 9–14 (in which it originated from the margins of old posttraumatic perforations), by cases 15 and 16 (where pieces of epithelium were apparently torn out of the TM and scattered into the ME), or by case 23 (where epithelium originating from the lining of the EEC was brought into the mastoid). In these instances, the transposed epithelium appears to constitute the source of origin of the cholesteatoma. And then again, infoldings of an injured TM and subsequent adhesions may be the source of epidermoid cysts within the TM itself (case 17) or lead to the formation of deep recesses and pockets (cases 18 and 21); these in turn could invite the development of a cholesteatoma (cases 19 and 20). Finally, when epithelium is hemmed in within a fracture cleft, it may, in the long run, start to proliferate (cases 28–29).

Posttraumatic cholesteatomata apparently occur more frequently than is indicated in the contemporary literature, which is largely confined to single case reports. *Eckel* [90] estimated its incidence as 0.4% of all longitudinal TB fractures. In the present material, the incidence was much higher, i.e. 5.7% of all longitudinal TB fractures, 6.1% of all injuries to the osseous walls of the EEC and of the tympanic cavity, and 2.6% following TM ruptures.

The figures just cited appear to show that the frequency of posttraumatic cholesteatoma is of an order of magnitude that has clinical relevance. Nevertheless, when seen in an overall context, cholesteatoma is still a rare, and usually late, complication of ME trauma.

The above case reports ought to have demonstrated that there is no typical ear (or skull) injury that predisposes to the formation of a cholesteatoma. It may develop on the basis of almost any kind of trauma that involves the ME.

The trauma evidently played only the role of a trigger. Additonal factors might come into play. Nevertheless, a wide fracture cleft in the EEC and injured canal skin may not be the only important cofactor as suggested by *Steurer* [418]. Retracted or pushed-in TM and also hemmed-in pieces of canal skin (that may be completely buried under an intact epithelium) may be of similar importance, as was suggested by some of the cases described above. Finally, one ought to recall that posttraumatic changes of the TM do not only occur in the presence of fractures.

It is not possible to decide on the basis of the present case material whether (a) a simultaneously present laceration of the ME mucosa [386] or a chronic inflammatory irritation [469] are important cofactors; (b) whether the trauma may activate a latent growth tendency of the epithelium, or (c) whether a posttraumatic tubal dysfunction plays a causative role, as was suggested by the above cases 30 and 31. At this point, these remain mere possibilities. Long-term observations of injured ears that receive no treatment at all should provide the necessary information; for obvious reasons, however, that is clinically not feasible. Therefore, further elucidation of these problems must mainly rely on studies in experimental animals.

7. Traumatic Lesions of the Round Window Membrane and Perilymphatic Fistulae

Knowledge about injuries to the RW membrane did not come about during the last 15 years, as a perusal of the contemporary literature might suggest. In 1897 already, *Barnick* [20] examined TB specimens histologically, obtained from victims of fatal head trauma. Finding sanguineous extravasates on the inside of the RW membrane, he saw their probable cause in labyrinthine pressure increases produced by the trauma. In his opinion, such increases would be rather slowly equilibrated via the aqueducts. Hence, they should affect the only place of the labyrinthine walls capable of yielding, i.e. the RW membrane.

Stenger [415] conducted experiments on rats, producing skull traumata by blows to their heads. In addition to other injuries, he found hemorrhages of varying extent in the RW region, in some cases even ruptured membranes. With respect to their causes, he concurred with *Barnick* [20]. *Wittmaack* [467] studied related problems, i.e. the effects of positive pressure pulses on the labyrinths of experimental animals. Yet, his attention was focused on the cochlear duct and not on the RW membrane.

Ulrich [443], in his histological studies on TB specimens after head trauma, found an RW membrane with fresh scars (his case XXII); however, his interpretation of the underlying mechanism differed from that of his predecessors. He stated that: 'The cochlear lumen is widest directly under the window. A transient deformation of the cochlea caused by a skull trauma must therefore exert the greatest strain on the soft tissues of this region.' This and other findings led him to the following conclusions: (1) perilymphatic pressure changes as such are not capable of rupturing the RW membrane, and (2) a torn RW membrane may heal spontaneously.

Brock [46] published his histological findings on an RW membrane ruptured 15 years earlier. A solid connective tissue mass had formed behind it, almost completely filling the lumen of the basal turn.

After these early, and rather detailed, descriptions, lesions of the RW membrane were hardly ever mentioned for the next several decades. The 1944 paper by *Kelemen* [230] on TB injuries, already mentioned, included a figure (his No. 78) showing an RW membrane with hemorrhagic infiltrations after head trauma, but the text did not elaborate on this case. *Schuknecht* [377] stated that RW membranes healed after injuries are frequently found, but he gave no further explanations. *Dietzel* [78] and *Fleischer* [118] independently described posttraumatic fissures of the labyrinthine capsule, especially in the region of the OW; but they did not describe the condition of the window itself nor did they mention perilymphatic leakage.

Simmons [400] in 1962 first established the concept of RW membrane lesions as a separate entity. He did not regard them as mere by-product of TB fractures. In experiments on cats, *Simmons* et al. [400] found the cochlear microphonics to decrease within a few hours after perforation of the RW membrane. The potentials usually recovered within the next 1–4 weeks. Postmortem histology showed repair of the injured membrane by scar tissue. Some further findings of his are also interesting, i.e. (a) that his animals displayed signs of vestibular disturbances, lasting for about 2 days, and (b) that in 2 animals the microphonics, for no apparent reasons, never recovered. In 1968, *Simmons* [398] reported corresponding clinical observations on 15 patients. They had suddenly lost their hearing and complained about spells of dizziness; these symptoms had first appeared after strenuous physical exercise. Based on the results of his own earlier animal experiments, he postulated that these symptoms might have been brought about by the rupture of a window membrane.

During the same year, *Fee* [109] reported on 3 patients with perilymphatic fistulae at the anterior margin of the stapes footplate. These fistulae had been produced by head trauma, and were detected during surgery. They had led to fluctuant hearing losses that progressively increased in severity. In addition, there were spells of vertigo that became aggravated when the patient laid down on the side of the involved ear. After surgical closure of the fistulae, the vertiginous attacks subsided, but the hearing did not recover.

Stroud and Calcaterra [421] reported on 4 more patients with perilymphatic fistulae at the anterior margin of the footplate. Some lesions had been produced by strenuous physical exercises, others by relatively mild head traumata. All 4 patients showed progressive high-tone hearing losses, complained about dizziness and displayed nystagmus of the paralytic type. In 3 patients, the vertigo disappeared after surgical closure of the fistula; in 2 of them, the hearing also improved.

Goodhill [141] operated on 3 patients, who had suffered sudden hearing losses after physical exercise. In 2 of them, he found perilymphatic fistulae both at the anterior margin of the stapes footplate and in the RW membrane, in the third patient only a rupture of the RW membrane. After closure of the fistulae, the hearing improved in 2 of the patients.

Freeman and Edmonds [129] observed ruptures of the RW membrane in 2 patients; they had experienced difficulties in air pressure equilibration while diving. Eventually, they became completely deaf in the involved ear. *Freeman* [130] called this an 'inner-ear barotrauma'.

The 1968 hypothesis of *Simmons* [398], i.e. that ruptures of the window membranes — the annular ligament and the RW membrane — might produce hearing losses and deafness, was thus confirmed by clinical and surgical observations. (The discussion will be continued in chapter 7.4.)

Since that time, a number of additional cases of posttraumatic, perilymphatic fistulae have been described so that a critical survey of their suspected causes as well as of their signs and symptoms might be in order. Nevertheless, since each author based his hypothesis about the modes of origin of these fistulae on his own collection of cases, clinical descriptions shall precede that discussion of the underlying pathophysiology.

7.1. Causes

From 42 published papers, 232 cases of perilymphatic fistulae were collected. Only those were included in which a membraneous defect in one or the other cochlear window (or a fracture or luxation of the stapes footplate) was demonstrated during surgery. Clinical cases, in which such conditions were merely suspected, were left out and likewise those in which the osseous labyrinthine walls had been directly injured. Further excluded were poststapedectomy fistulae because of the obvious impossibility to delimit the sequelae of a potential surgical trauma from the signs and symptoms produced by the fistula itself. As table LXXIII shows, most series were rather small, often limited to a single case, demonstrating the rarity of the entity under discussion.

When all reports are considered together, the incidence of perilymphatic leakage from either window was about equal. In 33 cases (14%), there were lesions of both windows. Bilateral ruptures of the RW membrane after barotrauma were observed by three authors. In 3 patients, perilymph was discharged through the TM ruptured by the same trauma; the condition had been diagnosed clinically. In 1 patient, a big surge of perilymph from the RW, ruptured behind an intact TM, was seen during surgery, suggesting an increased labyrinthine pressure [185].

Table LXXIII. Perilymphatic fistulae in the regions of the oval and round windows (literature survey)

Author	Fistula in oval window region	Fistulae in regions of both windows	Fistula in round window region	Remarks
Allam [4]	–	–	4	
Althaus [5]	5	–	1	
Arenberg et al. [12]	1	–	–	positive glycerol test
Behbehani and Kastenbauer [23]	2	–	–	
Boenninghaus and Gülzow [41]	–	–	4	
Chüden [59]	–	–	4	CSF discharge from the ear and TM perforation (once)
Cummings [66]	5	–	–	stapes luxation or fracture (5×)
Emmett et al. [96]	–	1	–	CSF discharge from EEC
Fee [109]	3	–	–	
Fernandes [111]	1	–	2	
Fraser and Harborow [128]	–	–	2	
Freeman [131, 132]	–	–	2	bilateral (once)
Friedman and Sassaki [136]	1	–	–	
Goodhill [142] *Goodhill* et al. [145]	24	19	4	
Goodman and Morioka [146]	–	–	1	
Gray and Barton [148]	–	3	5	
Grundfast and Bluestone [156]	3	–	2	craniostenosis (once)
Gunderson and Molvaer [166]	1	–	–	
Healy et al. [183, 184]	31	4	5	
Heermann et al. [185]	–	–	1	gusher
Howard [206]	1	–	–	CSF discharge from perforated TM
Jensma [215]	1	–	9	no location given in 2 cases
Kleinfeldt [244]	–	–	12	
Knight [251], *Knight and Phillips* [252]	–	–	7	bilateral (once)
Love and Waguespack [273]	12	6	4	in addition: 1 lateral transversal fracture

Table LXXIII. (cont.)

Lyons et al. [275]	–	–	2	
Maddox and Kosoy [284]	1	–	–	meningitis after 5 years
McNicoll [282]	–	–	1	TM perforation
Molvaer [306, 307]	1	–	1	
Montandon [309]	1	–	–	
Nedzelski and Barber [327]	–	–	4	
Pellegrini and de Firmas [342]	1	–	–	
Pullen [353]	–	–	3	
Riol et al. [54]	1	–	–	
Simmons [399]	2	–	1	
Stroud and Calcatterra [421]	4	–	–	
Taylor and Bicknell [426]	–	–	1	
Tonkin and Fagan [434]	–	–	13	bilateral (once)
Tyler [441]	–	–	2	
Total	102	33	97	3× bilateral RW ruptures 4× CSF discharge from ear

232 (+ 2 of unknown location)

The presumed causes of fistulae, if and when provided by the author, are listed in table LXXIV and the incidences of the three main signs and symptoms of fistulae found in various locations in table LXXV later on. (The names of individual authors are only given when there were some special findings.)

The places of 33 combined injuries, both of the OW and the RW, are listed as 'unknown'; likewise 2 other cases, in which the places of leakage could not be determined [215]. Finally, there were a number of papers in which neither a trauma was mentioned nor the location of the fistula given.

The causes listed are essentially the same as those that produce rupture of the TM (cf. chapter 3.1) and ossicular injuries (cf. chapter 4.1). One additional cause was suspected by some authors [176, 273], i.e. there might be a congenital weakness of, or an already existing perforation in, the regions of the footplate or of the RW. These authors supported their assumptions by stating either that their findings had been made in children who had not yet suffered an adequate trauma (the first sign of illness being an otogenic

Table LXXIV. Causes of 234 perilymphatic fistulae collected from the literature

Percent of total	Cause	Number of cases	Location		
			oval window	round window	unknown
6	congenital	13	5	8	–
18	blunt skull trauma	43	10	8	25
3	transtympanal injury	7	4	1	2
	slap on the ear,	5	1	1	3
6	explosion	3	1	1	1
	acoustic trauma	6	–	4	2
	increased intra-	52	5	6	41
40	thoracic pressure,				
	barotrauma	37	4	20	13
	anesthesia	4	1	3	–
2	various other causes	5	2	2	1
25	unknown	59	2	17	40

meningitis [273] or a labyrinthitis [156]), or that a substantial malformation had already existed in the region of either window [156].

The category 'intrathoracic pressure' in table LXXIV includes everything that may produce pressure elevations, such as coughing, laughing, blowing one's nose, lifting of heavy loads, etc. In some cases, it was not even clear whether or not the Eustachian tubes were ventilated during these activities. Under the entry 'anesthesia', 1 case is listed in which a mask was employed (possibly facilitating a passive tubal inflation), and 3 other cases in which intubation had been used.

The category 'other causes', includes some individual observations: one fistula of the OW incurred after irrigation of the ear canal [23]; a second one was seen after an upper respiratory infection [5]; one fistula of the RW was found 4 years after an injury by a welding spark [273]; another in an ear in which a radical mastoidectomy had been performed 14 years earlier [59]; finally, fistulae of both windows that had followed gunshot injuries [96].

Inspection of table LXXIV reveals that nearly one half of all RW ruptures were produced by pressure changes, either sudden (6%) or protracted ones (40%). In second place are the unknown causes (25%), i.e. those cases in which perilymphatic leakage was demonstrated, although no trauma could be identified. In this category, delineation from congenital defects is uncertain, and classification by the author in question in one or another category was arbitrary to some degree. Blunt head trauma occupied third place, followed by the relatively rare direct injuries, i.e. transtympanal or iatrogenic ones.

Only a few of the modes of injury listed appeared to prefer one or the other window. Obviously, transtympanal injuries rarely involved the RW, which is well protected behind the promontory lip. On the other hand, the RW was more easily injured by air pressure changes, i.e. either in the form of an acoustic trauma or of a barotrauma, than the OW. All other causes involved the two windows with about equal frequency.

7.2. Signs, Symptoms and Their Diagnostic Significance

The signs and symptoms of perilymphatic fistulae vary considerably. Classical descriptions [109, 132, 144] mention a sudden onset of pain in the ear and the feeling as if something had burst within it; thereafter, fullness in the ear is experienced and sometimes bubbling noises are perceived. Later on, there are fluctuant hearing losses, tinnitus and spells of dizziness. These signs and symptoms are precisely those of Menière's disease. The following case may be cited as an example: a 10-year-old girl had displayed signs and symptoms of the kind mentioned for a period of 2 years. On the basis of a positive glycerol test, the diagnosis of Menière's disease was made. A subsequent tympanoscopy, however, revealed a fistula at the anterior margin of the footplate [12].

Many cases were described, in which the initial symptoms were not that obvious; one of the three main symptoms was missing, or there was nothing but a hearing loss or dizziness. (A surgical exploration, solely on account of tinnitus, was apparently never done.) *Pullen* [353] expressed the opinion that hearing loss, not dizzy spells, is the only characteristic sign of a perilymphatic fistula. On the other hand, *Healy* et al. [183] stressed the occurrence of dizzy spells and unsteadiness and considered the hearing loss an inconstant sign.

Table LXXV presents the incidence of the three main signs and symptoms: hearing loss, tinnitus and dizziness. Once more, there is a large-sized category labeled 'location unknown'; in several of the papers surveyed only the signs and symptoms were listed, but not the place of the fistula.

As indicated in the last line of table LXXV, some hearing loss was nearly always present. In only 12 cases (5%), hearing was listed as normal or, expressed more accurately, the audiogram had not changed in relation to one taken before there were any specific complaints. Tinnitus was present in approximately one half of all cases and dizzy spells occurred in about three quarters of them.

Table LXXV. Incidence of hearing loss, dizziness and tinnitus in perilymphatic fistulae: oval and round window locations (percentages given in parentheses)

Location	Hearing loss	Dizziness	Tinnitus	Combination of all three symptoms
Oval window region	43	39	11	10
(n = 46)	(94)	(75)	(24)	(22)
Round window region	75	44	31	27
(n = 79)	(95)	(66)	(39)	(34)
Oval and round window	10	9	3	3
region (n = 10)	(100)	(90)	(30)	(30)
Location unknown	94	88	70	69
(n = 99)	(95)	(89)	(71)	(70)
Total	222	170	115	109
(n = 234)	(95)	(73)	(49)	(47)

The signs and symptoms, when listed according to the various fistula locations, were rather evenly distributed. Hence, it was not possible to correlate a given sign or symptom with a specific place of lesion, in an effort to differentiate fistulae in the RW region from those in the OW region.

Detailed audiological examinations give contradictory results. Reports included low-tone losses [399], high-tone losses [434] as well as flat losses [136]. Combined conductive and sensorineural losses were also seen [59, 66, 96, 183, 342]. If present, fluctuant hearing losses, as a rule, increased gradually in severity [109, 127, 132, 146, 421]. *Simmons* [399], however, mentioned that the hearing loss might also slowly improve. Several authors pointed out that, quite often, there is a relatively large loss for speech discrimination in the presence of a mild pure-tone loss [109, 183, 184, 273]. The incidences of the various forms and degrees of hearing loss reported were as follows:

		%
Normal hearing	12	5
Fluctuant hearing loss	32	14
Mild to moderate sensorineural hearing loss	76	32
Severe sensorineural hearing loss and complete deafness	114	49
Total	234	100

Impedance audiometry was not very helpful either. *Love and Wague-spack* [278] found the results ambiguous, provided there was not a concurrent injury of the ossicular chain. *Goodman and Morioka* [146] observed in 1 case an increase in conductance. *Althaus* (in discussing the paper by *Goodman and Morioka* [146]) warned against impedance audiometry when a fistula is suspected because of the danger of further damaging the labyrinth.

Vestibular examinations, likewise, did not give unequivocal results. Among 170 patients complaining of dizzy spells, 36 (21%) showed spontaneous nystagmus; in 10 of them, it was of the paralytic type (i.e. toward the normal ear) and in 11 others of the excitatory type (i.e. toward the involved ear). *Stroud and Calcaterra* [421], in 1 patient, observed a change in direction: originally, there was an excitatory nystagmus, later on a paralytic one. Positional nystagmus was occasionally seen when the patient was lying on the involved ear [5, 109, 156, 421]. Some found this sign rather frequently (in 4 out of 15 cases [142]; in 33 of 40 cases [183]). The importance of the various walking tests and of the Romberg test was also stressed, the Romberg being positive in 20 out of 40 cases [183].

Positive fistula signs have been described [5, 109, 156]. Some found them rather frequently (in 15 of 40 patients [183]; in 7 of 12 patients [273]). *Grundfast and Bluestone* [156] detected a positive fistula sign in 1 patient who did not complain about dizziness. *Nedzelski and Barber* [327] observed dizzy attacks evoked by Valsalva maneuvers in 2 patients. *Spitzer and Ritter* [410] found a Tullio phenomenon in a patient with a fracture that ran across the promontory between the two windows and was discharging perilymph.

Opinions about the results of caloric stimulation are also divided. *Love and Waguespack* [278] found reduced excitability in 62% (i.e. in 8 of 13 patients); *Healy* et al. [183], however, in only 25%. The latter authors did not consider ENG helpful for the diagnosis of perilymphatic fistulae on account of its large variability, an opinion shared by *Goodhill* et al. [145]. *Althaus* (discussion remark to *Goodman and Morioka* [146]), once more, considered caloric stimulation potentially harmful, since it might damage the labyrinth.

Other specific methods of examination were hardly ever mentioned. The glycerol test was employed once, but there was a false-positive result [12]. No reports were published that included pathological X-ray findings. *Gray and Barton* [148] demonstrated the cochlear aqueduct by means of polycyclic tomography, suspecting it to be abnormally wide; the results were inconclusive.

Fee [109] suggested to apply radioisotopes intrathecally and subsequently to measure their activity in the ME. In this manner, he thought, the transfer of CSF into the perilymph and its discharge via the fistula might be demonstrated. *Stroud and Calcaterra* [421], following up on this suggestion, injected albumen marked with techneticum in 1 patient, but did not demonstrate any positive results. *Emmett* et al. [96], on the other hand, applied indium-diethylenetriaminepentaacetic acid (DTPA) intrathecally in a patient with suspected injuries of both windows; 24 h later, they were able to prove its presence in gelfoam sponges they had put onto the windows. This is the only case published so far in which a perilymphatic fistula was demonstrated by means of scintillography.

On the basis of the reported findings, one has to conclude that it is not yet feasible to secure the diagnosis of a perilymphatic fistula clinically — not even to make it reasonably probable. An adequate trauma cannot be proven in every case. The triad, hearing loss, tinnitus and vertigo, cannot be used to differentiate a fistula from Menière's disease; and if the vertigo is missing the clinical picture is essentially the same as that of a sudden hearing loss. Therefore, when suspecting a fistula, one should explore the ME surgically in an effort to either prove or disprove one's suspicion. Therapeutic measures, if required, can be taken in the same session.

7.3. Therapy and Its Results

Spontaneous self-repair of ruptured window membranes occurs quite readily. *Ulrichs'* [443] postmortem findings of an RW membrane closed over by scar tissue (his case XXII) were already mentioned. In experiments on cats, *Bellucci and Wolff* [26] were able to demonstrate membraneous closure of the *OW* within 3 days after stapes extraction. *Simmons* et al. [400], likewise on cats, observed spontaneous closure of experimentally ruptured *RW* membranes.

Chvojka and Mrovek [61] saw 2 patients with stapes subluxations. The dehiscences had been closed over by scar tissue. RW membranes repaired by scar tissue were found in several patients operated on the suspicion of a fistula (1 case [4]; 1 case [23]; 5 cases [41]; 1 case [321]). *Simmons* [399] as well as *Goodhill* [144] were of the opinion that the majority of ruptured windows close spontaneously. For patients with suspectd ruptures, they advised strict bed rest with the head elevated by 30°; abdominal pressing should be avoided so as not to elevate the perilymphatic pressure, which might endanger the spontaneous repair. Surgical exploration of the ME was recommended only if the signs and symptoms had not been alleviated within 10 days. *Tonkin and Fagan* [434] essentially concurred with this opinion, although they chose to intervene surgically already after 3–4 days. (Earlier, *Goodhill* [143] had made the same recommendation.) *Healy* et al. [183] as well as *Pullen* [353] preferred early surgery.

It is the consensus of opinion that a firm diagnosis is not possible without surgical exploration. The clinical evidence for the spontaneous closure of ruptured windows is considered as rather weak. Be that as it may, the following series of reports on surgically proven spontaneous closures does not strike an optimistic note: In 5 patients the deafness persisted [41]; 1 patient retained a hearing loss [327]; 1 other patient continued to be dizzy [4]; it was in only 1 case that the inner-ear functions were completely restored [23].

The *surgical approach* is rather uniform: The posterior part of the tympanic cavity is uncovered by raising a tympanomeatal flap. If required, a portion of the lateral attic wall is taken down to expose the OW, exactly as in a stapedectomy procedure. A number of authors recommended to reduce the promontory lip over the RW niche to expose fully the membrane [5, 109, 141, 327, 434]. Thereafter, perilymphatic discharge may already be noticed. It may be synchronized with the respiratory cycle. Occasionally, there is a surge of fluid [185, 342].

If discharge cannot be observed, *Goodhill* [141] suggested to lyse the fibrous strands that are frequently present over a fistula and then, after drying the membrane thoroughly by means of gelfoam sponges, to observe it continuously for about 20 min under ×25 magnification for the possible reappearance of fluid. Discharge might also be provoked by carefully pressing on the incudostapedial joint [144] or by elevating the intracranial pressure, e.g. by lowering the head or by performing the test of Queckenstedt [143, 156, 183]. It was only in rare cases that a defect of the RW membrane was found without any discharge of perilymph, or that the scala tympani appeared to be dry behind a perforation [244].

If one disregards stapedial subluxations [66] or footplate fractures [273, 342], defects in the OW region were almost always located in the area of the *fissula ante fenestram*. As just mentioned, *Goodhill* [143] frequently saw fibrous strands more or less obscuring the region of the fistula. He believed that they might be the result of futile attempts at spontaneous closure. During histological examination of a footplate defect, *Healy* et al. [184] were able to demonstrate granulations around the fistula. Others [41, 244, 434] saw slitlike tears in the RW membrane with freely floating margins, or sometimes roundish defects of various sizes with thickened rims, not unlike those of old TM perforations. Occasionally, a dehiscence cannot be detected; *Goodhill* [143] is of the opinion that in such cases hidden marginal defects might be present.

Some authors recommend stapedectomy for the management of peri-lymphatic fistulae in the OW region [66, 109, 184]. Most writers, however, prefer to simply freshen up the wound margins carefully and to cover the defect with a free autologous graft (fat tissue, connective tissue, fascia, peri-chondrium or vein grafts). For the postsurgical period, several authors order strict bed rest with the head elevated, laxatives to avoid abdominal pressing and prophylactive dosages of antibiotics [96, 132, 141, 184, 434].

Fistulae occasionally reoccur after surgical closure as is shown in the following tabulation:

Love and Waguespack [273]	3 cases (1 additional case with granuloma formation in the RW region and persisting vertigo)
Healy et al. [184]	2 cases
Pullen [353]	1 case
Fee [109]	1 case
Tonkin and Fagan [434]	1 case
Chüden [59]	1 case that recurred twice

Since in the cases of *Love and Waguespack* [273] and in that of *Tonkin and Fagan* [434] the fistulae recurred when fat tissue was being employed, these authors do not recommend its use anymore.

The functional result of successful closures of fistulae are presented in table LXXVI, as far as they could be collected from the literature. Cases in which cochlear functions were normal prior to surgery are not listed.

Combined injuries as well as those for which the paper in question did not present a clear correlation between location and clinical findings are once more listed in the 'unknown' category. With respect to the audiometric findings, 'return to normal' and mere 'improvements' are listed separately. Vertigo and tinnitus do not permit such fine gradations.

As table LXXVI indicates, it was mainly the vertigo that was improved after surgery (in 98%). With 75% improvement, tinnitus was next in order. Auditory improvements were achieved in only 48% of all cases, return to normal hearing levels in a mere 15%. The auditory results, moreover, appeared to depend on the duration of the postsurgical observation, i.e. progressive improvements occurred over relatively long periods of observation, i.e. up to 4 months [215, 282]. And then again, in 2 patients transient, post-

Table LXXVI. Perilymphatic fistulae: postsurgical results for the locations in either window region (percentages given in parentheses)

Location	Total number of cases (= 100%)	Return to normal	Improved	Unchanged	Made worse
A. Hearing loss					
OW region	26	7 (27)	11 (42)	8 (31)	–
RW region	66	14 (21)	23 (35)	28 (42)	1 (2)
Unknown	127	11 (9)	40 (31)	71 (56)	5 (4)
Subtotal	219	32 (15)	74 (33)	107 (49)	6 (3)
B. Vertigo					
OW region	24		24 (100)	–	–
RW region	34		33 (97)	1 (3)	–
Unknown	68		66 (97)	2 (3)	–
Subtotal	126		123 (98)	3 (2)	–
C. Tinnitus					
OW region	8		7 (88)	1 (12)	–
RW region	25		23 (92)	2 (8)	–
Unknown	42		26 (62)	15 (36)	1 (2)
Subtotal	75		56 (75)	18 (24)	1 (1)

surgical improvements were observed, followed by renewed deterioration to presurgical levels [156].

For all three entities, hearing loss, tinnitus and vertigo, the postsurgical results were not seen to depend on which of the two windows had been ruptured. The success rates were about equal for both windows.

The improvements of tinnitus and vertigo did not appear to vary with the time interval between the window rupture and surgery. However, several authors are of the opinion that the earlier surgery is performed, the better the auditory results that may be expected. Boenninghaus and Gülzow [41] set the limit at 7 days, Goodhill [142] at 13 days, and Healy et al. [183] at 3 weeks. Some reports can only be partly evaluated in this respect, since the necessary details were not given. Goodhill [142], for example, simply lists 26 poor auditory results for intervals between 15 days and several years, Love and Waguespack [273] 15 for intervals between 6 months and 29 years. A summary of the results that could be evaluated is presented in table LXXVII.

Table LXXVII. Perilymphatic fistulae: the effect of the time interval between the trauma and surgery on the auditory results

Auditory results	Distribution			
	number of cases	min	max	median
Return to normal	15	2 days	to 18 months	10 days
Improved	34	1 day	to 13 years	10 days
Unchanged	31	1 day	to 8 years	6 weeks

Inspection of table LXXVII shows that one cannot really set a firm time limit because of the considerable variations in all three categories. There was no difference in this respect between complete returns to normal hearing and mere improvements. However, if one plots the auditory results (improvements or the lack thereof) against the time intervals between trauma and surgery a correlation becomes apparent. In figure 10, results are grouped in five time intervals. Plotted in semilog fashion, the five points lie reasonably close to a straight line, with time zero representing 100%. Even if one realizes that these results rest on the evaluation of only 80 patients, i.e. on one third of all published cases, figure 10 strongly suggests that the probability of postsurgical auditory improvements decreases exponentially with the interval between trauma and surgery. As already said, there is no absolute time limit for surgical intervention in patients with perilymphatic fistulae. Nevertheless, one should make every attempt to operate as early as possible, since that provides the best chance of restoring auditory function.

7.4. Rupture of the Cochlear Windows: Pathophysiological Considerations

The structures that are subject to the type of ruptures under discussion must be desribed first, i.e. the annular ligament of the stapes and the membrane of the RW.

The asymmetrical arrangement of the *annular ligament* was already mentioned in chapter 4.2. At its anterior margin, the fibers are longer and thinner (diameter: 300 μm) than those at the posterior margin (diameter: 500 μm) [26, 49]. Furthermore, the ligament is said to be more compliant at the upper and lower margins than at the anterior and posterior margins [6]. The

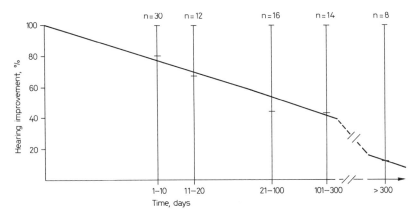

Fig. 10. Perilymphatic fistulae: hearing improvement with time between injury and surgery. Time in log intervals. Data collected from the literature.

fissula ante fenestram is thought to represent an (additional) *locus minoris resistentiae* [6, 144]. The clinical findings agree rather well with these structural details. In the majority of cases cited in the preceding chapters, the preferred place of perilymphatic fistulae — provided it was listed — was at the anterior margin.

The *RW* lies at the posterior end of the promontory in an almost horizontal plane in a deep niche formed by an osseous lip of the promontory and the subiculum. By virtue of its position, it usually cannot be seen, even when viewed from the EEC. Frequently, moreover, the entrance to the niche is almost occluded by mucous membrane folds (in 55% [419]), some of which may be touching the window. The window membrane itself is about 20 μm thick [302]; its anterior portion is curved in superior direction so as to duplicate the turn of scala tympani, which it terminates. It yields passively to cochlear fluid displacements [488]. The circumference of the membrane forms a trapezoid, rather than a ring; its posterior width is 2.8 mm, its anterior width 1.4 mm and its (horizontal) length 1.5 mm [419]. In the medial wall of scala tympani lies the orifice of the cochlear aqueduct at a distance of 0.3 mm from the window and hidden behind a small bony spur, the *crista semilunaris* [337].

The membrane consists of three strata: on the tympanal side, ther is epithelium, one or two layers thick [270], carrying goblet cells at the periphery [359]. It is a direct continuation of th ME mucosa [226]. The *tunica propria* below it consists of large numbers of collagen fibers. It can be mechanically stressed. The elastic fibers described [270] appear to belong mainly to the numerous capillaries present [435]. The (collagen) fibers run chiefly in radial directions, connecting directly with the fibers of Sharpey at the osseous rim. Both at the center and at the periphery of the *tunica propria* are thin layers of circular fibers [270]. The nerve fibers supplying this stratum originate from the tympanic plexus [197, 226]. The innermost stratum of the membrane is an endothelium, one cell thick; it is part of the perilymphatic lining of scala tympani [25, 226]. Capillaries are found on top of this layer [359]. The epithelium of the window appears to be less transparent to the beam of the electron microscope than that covering the adjacent bone [25, 126]. *Arnold and von Ilberg* [14] showed, on the basis of dye experiments, that perilymph, when under pressure, may seep into the subepithelial layers of the RW membrane and from there into the lymphatic spaces of the ME.

Kobrak [254] studied the displacement of isolated RW membranes obtained from fresh human cadavers. He employed a kymographic method, making use of a small mirror glued onto the membrane. For dc pressures of up to 50 cm H_2O, displacements occurred symmetrically in both directions and the relation between pressure and displacement was linear. If the membrane had remained in situ, however, the outwardly directed displacements were larger than those directed inward.

Ivarsson and Petersen [212] conducted such experiments on TB preparations with the RW membrane kept in situ. By means of a capillary cemented into the superior canal, they measured shifts in inner-ear fluid, in terms of the volume displaced, in response to increases in dc pressure, which they applied at various places. When forcing the RW membrane by changing the pressure in a small, airtight chamber built over the niche, they obtained the following results: Outward shifts and inward shifts were almost equal. At +20 cm H_2O, for example, the volume shift was +0.12 μl and, at −20 cm H_2O, −12 μl. The resulting pressure/volume-shift characteristic was S-shaped, i.e. strongly nonlinear. At p> ±20 cm H_2O, the volume shifts began to level off at ±0.12 μl, asymptotically approaching a maximum. Measurements were carried out up to ±70 cm H_2O, but a true plateau was never reached. For the stapes footplate, the pressure/volume-shift characteristic was similarly shaped. However, with the ossicular chain intact, maximal volume shifts were only between +0.02 and −0.03 μl. With the chain interrupted, shifts were of the same order of magnitude as those measured at the RW. Thus, stapedial displacements are not really limited by the stiffness of the annular ligament, but rather by that of the ME structures, as older measurements had suggested [350].

Densert et al. [68a] obtained similar results in cats. They did not measure volume shifts, but rather the alterations in labyrinthine pressure in response to pressure changes in the EEC. *Densert* et al. [68b] were able to show in preparations of *human* TB that an increased labyrinthine pressure, while displacing the stapes in an outward direction, affects the ME impedance. Such changes could be directly assessed in patients.

(It must be noted, however, that results derived from cadaver experiments often deviate, both quantitatively as well as qualitatively, from those obtained during life, e.g. values of ME impedance [502], of basilar membrane displacements [498], or of RW displacements [497]. Therefore, the above results must be viewed with some caution.)

In *live* cats, the inner-ear impedance was assessed. It was calculated as the ratio of SPL to velocity of the RW displacement, the latter being measured with a laser kymograph [497]. When high-level signals (SPL > 135 dB) were suddenly switched on, the inner-ear impedance increased with the signal level, although in a rather erratic manner. This type of reaction was never observed after sacrifice of the animal; then, the impedance remained independent of signal level, as was to be expected. When responding to the high SPL mentioned, the RW was seen to abruptly shift its resting position, but once more only in live cats. This phenomenon, apparently protective in nature, was attributed to alterations of the endolymph/perilymph pressure (or volume) ratios, perhaps mediated by changes in CSF or blood pressure [497].

Kleinfeldt and Dahl [245], once more in cadaver ears, tested the pressure resistance of the RW membrane, which they were able to displace up to ±0.12 mm. When the pressure increase reached about 4 kPa (approximately 30 mm Hg), the membrane ruptured, usually at its margins; central perforations occurred less frequently. *Miriszlai and Sandor* [303] conducted similar experiments in cat ears. When using the above technique, they never saw fistulae developing in the *OW*. The *RW* membrane yielded at 23 ± 17 mm Hg, with actual values varying between 6 and 66 mm Hg. Occasionally, the membrane did not rupture even at pressures of up to 230 mm Hg, although the experimenters gained the impression that in such cases perilymph kept seeping into the submucosal tissues of the RW niche in the manner originally described by *Arnold and von Ilberg* [14].

Axelsson et al. [16] in a study on guinea pigs, determined the fate of RW membranes after their experimental rupture. Of 13 animals, which were kept for various periods of time (9–95 days) before sacrifice, the membrane had healed in 12; in most of them, scars could not be seen macroscopically. The only perforation still persisting was found on the tenth postoperative day. In their experiments on cats that were already described, *Simmons* et al. [400] had obtained similar results. *Stewart and Belal* [419] reported histological findings on a human RW membrane, torn in the course of a transversal fracture. (They did not give the interval between trauma and death.) Their illustration shows osseous obliteration of the basal portion of scala tympani and wound margins thickened by scarring. They appeared to be epithelialized, displaying no further tendency to heal.

The cause of transmeatal injuries is self-evident and needs no discussion. Poststapedectomy fistulae will not be discussed either. In the opinion of *Goodhill* [144] and of *Althaus* [6], either window could be ruptured 'explosively' or 'implosively' under the effect of a head trauma or a barotrauma, respectively. There might also be what *Althaus* called 'spontaneous fistulae', i.e. membranes torn by a trivial trauma, apparently after having been weakened by some undefined (or unknown) factor.

These authors regarded ruptures as 'explosive' when produced by a sudden increase in endocranial pressure (e.g. due to a head trauma). The pressure pulse was thought to be transmitted via the cochlear aqueduct into the perilymphatic fluid (possibly also along the nerve fibers from the inner meatus through the spiral tractus foraminosus, the endolymphatic duct and the vestibular aqueduct). This, in their opinion, would lead to a sudden displacement of the window membranes and, consequently, to their rupture.

Authors regarded ruptures as 'implosive' when produced by a sudden pressure increase in the EEC (e.g. by a blow to the head or sudden exposure to a high-level sound) or in the ME (e.g. due to a Valsalva maneuver). Moreover, in the opinion of *Althaus* [6], an impaired patency of the cochlear aqueduct should pose a special danger when windows are ruptured 'implosively', since there would be no possibility to equalize the pressure via that channel. (All these considerations are quite hypothetical. The entire subject will be discussed in more detail in chapter 7.8.)

Before considering the other causes mentioned one must first discuss all pathological conditions of the window membranes that may exist and elucidate the patency of the cochlear aqueduct.

Congenital defects at the anterior margin of the stapes footplate have been described, with discharge of perilymph and entrance of pathogens through this opening [27, 404]; likewise, there are malformations of the RW, in which the membrane is replaced by bone [332].

Gussen [167] described a loose tissue, rich in melanocytes, that she found in the RW niche, nearly always in fetuses, less frequently during later life. Because of its similar appearance, she believes that it is related to the arachnoidal tissue in the orifice of the cochlear aqueduct. Her finding might provide evidence for the origin of tissue bridges that are frequently found lying across the RW membrane (cf. above [141]).

Stewart and Belal [419] described the migration of pus through an RW membrane altered by an ME infection. In other cases, they frequently found thickening of the membrane and sometimes its obliteration by scar tissue. *Knight* [251] thought such membrane alterations were produced by infections and might represent the causes of RW defects he had observed in children. RW membranes altered by scar tissue were accidentally found during surgery by several authors [4, 23, 41]. *Nedzelski and Barber* [327] reported a window rupture that occurred 14 years after a trauma originally caused by an explosion; the lesion was accompanied by a transient hearing loss. Authors suspected that an old scar had yielded under the effect of a trivial trauma. As demonstrated by these findings, the existence of weak spots in the RW membrane must be accepted as fact.

Notions about the structure and function of the cochlear aqueduct vary rather widely. This channel, running through bone and lined by dura, is 10–14 mm in length. It has a funnel-shaped orifice at the posterior surface of the petrous bone, 0.5–1.25 mm in diameter; but it narrows considerably toward scala tympani, where its opening is only 0.05–0.125 mm wide [11, 354]. This orifice is close to the RW membrane, as was already mentioned. The duct connects the subarachnoidal space with the perilymphatic space.

Winkler [465] maintained that the aqueduct is occluded by an inverted, blind sack, consisting of arachnoidal tissue. *Tainmont and Uitenhoef* [425] believed that the duct is a phylogenetic remnant, without function, and is frequently closed. *Anson and Donaldson* [11] described it as being filled with loose connective tissue which would permit the passage of fluid. *Nishimura* et al. [330] confirmed the latter finding by electron microscopy in guinea pigs. *Rask-Anderson* et al. [354] found the duct closed by bone in 3 out of 82 human TB specimens. *Palva and Dammert* [337] were of the opinion that the aqueduct is always patent, but that the presence of side channels as well as histological sectioning in a tangential manner occasionally gives the false impression that the duct might be closed. Yet, the same authors admitted that, under the effect of inflammations, the connective tissue within the canal could swell, effectively cutting off the subarachnoidal space from the perilymphatic one.

Waltner [454] described a barrier membrane in the labyrinthine opening of the aqueduct, consisting of a single-cell layer in continuity with the endothelium of scala tympani. However, he did not think that this membrane could withstand mechanical stresses and, therefore, that it would not constitute a true barrier. He believed that the reticular tissue within the aqueduct and the corpora amylacea contained in it could buffer pressure pulses of the central nervous system (CNS) fluid which, otherwise, might rupture the RW membrane. *Palva and Dammert* [337] found such a barrier membrane in only 2 of 20 TB specimens. *Spector* et al. [408], on the other hand, confirmed its regular existence. Nevertheless, these authors believed that the aqueduct, as a rule, is freely patent, since they found erythrocytes in scala tympani of several postmortem specimens obtained from children with intracerebral hemorrhages. *Wlodyka* [468], finally, conducted dye studies and made casts of the canal. He concluded that the duct is always patent in fetuses, but that it frequently becomes narrower with increasing age. Beyond the age of 60, it was patent in only 30% of his specimens.

The patency of the aqueduct was demonstrated in *functional* studies conducted in experimental animals. In guinea pigs, *Kleinschmidt and Vick* [246] found that, after some perilymph was withdrawn, it was replaced by CSF. Their result was based on the analysis of perilymphatic proteins. *Kobrak* [253] demonstrated in rabbits that pressure changes in the CSF spaces produced corresponding labyrinthine volume alterations, but *with a temporal delay and of a relatively small magnitude.* (As will be explained in chapter 7.8, these two features are typical for the underlying mechanism.) *Ahlén* [2], also experimenting on rabbits, saw variations in the hight of the perilymphatic fluid column in experimentally produced fistulae; for example, it varied synchronously with the respiratory cycle. Furthermore, he found the perilymphatic pressure to rise when a mechanical pressure was exerted on the atlanto-occipital membrane or the thorax.

Kerth and Allen [234] measured in cat an increase in perilymphatic pressure produced by a rise in intracranial pressure. They also observed perilymphatic pressure variations sychronized with the respiratory cycle. After occlusion of the aqueduct, these became smaller, but did never completely vanish. *Densert* et al. [68a] found experimentally induced perilymphatic pressure increments to diminish slowly, presumably by the release of fluid via the aqueduct.

Miriszlai and Sandor [303], also in cat experiments, were able to increase the perilymphatic pressure, maximally by 5.8 mm Hg, by letting the head dangle or by compressing the thorax. They saw bulging of the RW membrane in 70% of their animals and its rupture in 40%. *Carlborg* [52] obtained similar results. He raised the perilymphatic pressure by compressing the neck veins, by increasing the body fluids, by letting the head dangle, or by inducing hypercapnia or hypoxia. Decreases in blood pressure were followed by a decline in perilymphatic pressure.

For obvious reasons, such functional tests can hardly be conducted in man. Nevertheless, a patent aqueduct must be presumed to exist in those patients, in whom, after opening the labyrinth (during stapedectomy, for example), fluid is discharged in copious amounts and for quite a long time; this is referred to as a pressure-labyrinth or a gusher. The incidence of this event was given as 1:1,000 or 1:2,000 [185] or even as high as 1:300 [309]. *Gray and Barton* [148], while accidentally finding a ruptured RW membrane during surgery, saw variations in the perilymphatic level synchronized with the respiratory cycle. Increased discharge of perilymph through a ruptured window could be provoked either by letting the head dangle or by executing the test of Queckenstedt [156, 183]. As was already mentioned, *Emmet* et al. [96] found indium-111-DTPA to be transmitted from the CSF space into the perilymphatic space. *Myers* [323] was able to demonstrate a rise in perilymphatic pressure in monkey and in man after compressing both jugular veins and thus increasing the intracranial pressure.

These results indicate that the connection between the perilymphatic space and the subarachnoidal space is patent in the majority of humans, although, as a rule, the duct is apparently quite narrow and permits only a slow transfer of fluid; notice the rarity of the gusher phenomenon and the long time delay in the experiments of *Kobrak* [253].

Even though perilymphatic fistulae usually produce characteristic clinical signs and symptoms, the information about the specific lesions they may create in the inner-ear sense organs is conflicting.

Weisskopf et al. [460], in experiments on guinea pigs, found cochlear microphonic losses of a mere 6–8 dB after rupturing the RW membrane. They concluded that a perilymphatic fistula as such does not appreciably affect the auditory function.

Simmons et al. [400], as will be recalled, saw microphonic losses persisting in some of their animals following spontaneous closure of RW perforations. Some of his clinical patients, moreover, became completely deaf after the RW membrane had been ruptured by increases in intracranial pressure [401]. Based on these two observations, *Simmons* [399] advanced the notion of a 'double-membrane break', reasoning that the same event responsible for the window rupture might, on occasion, rupture one of the intracochlear membranes, usually Reissner's membrane. This in turn would lead to a mixing of perilymph and endolymph, causing a critical loss of the cochlear resting potentials and producing grave changes in both end organs [399]. Hence, in *Simmons'* opinion, the window rupture would not be the direct cause of the observed functional losses, but simply one of two (or several) concurrent events. In most cases, surgical closure of the window might not be required. More important would be strict bed rest, which should aid spontaneous healing. *Goodhill* [144] concurred with this opinion. *Gussen* [168] was able to demonstrate healed ruptures of Reissner's membrane histologically in 2 human TB.

Axelsson et al. [16], in their experiments on guinea pigs already mentioned, obtained contrary findings. After experimentally rupturing the RW membrane, they observed all transitions between normal electrocochlear responses and their complete extinction. Histologically, they saw lesions of the stria vascularis as well as hemorrhages into the perilymphatic space and, in 4 animals, degeneration of the organ of Corti. These histological findings were well correlated with the electrophysiological results. Ruptures of the *intra*cochlear membranes were never observed.

Finally, there is a single clinical case report by *Azem and Caldarelli* [17]. Their patient, after blowing his nose rather forcefully, experienced a hearing loss, tinnitus and transient spells of dizziness. The hearing loss was of the combined type. During surgery, a fractured footplate was found; perilymph had seeped through the fracture gap under the mucosal covering of the footplate, but had not entered the free ME space. Following the replacement of the stapes by a prosthesis, the clinical signs and symptoms subsided.

The two last-mentioned observations indicate that there is a definite causal relation between the pathological discharge of perilymph from the labyrinthine space via a fistula and the observed inner-ear signs and symptoms.

7.5. Our Clinical Results

In our own patient material, a total of 8 perilymphatic fistulae in the region of the OW had occurred after *stapedectomy*. In some of these patients, the surgery had been performed several years earlier. These lesions are only mentioned in passing, but will not be discussed further, since they do not actually belong in the class of posttraumatic changes.

In 4 patients, *lateral transversal* fractures were seen to run across both cochlear windows and the annular ligament and the RW membrane were torn. Because of the promontory fractures and because of the grave damage that had most likely occurred in the inner ear, no reconstructive measures were undertaken. The defects in the labyrinthine wall were covered only in an effort to prevent ascending infections. When necessary, the FN was decompressed. Clinical details on these 4 cases were given in chapter 5.4 on TB fractures. Here, they are only brought up once more because of the window lesions incurred.

7.5.1. Case Reports

Isolated window ruptures had occurred in 15 patients. On account of the small number, a summarizing table would not serve any useful purpose. Therefore, each individual case will be briefly described:

Case 1. Female, 46 years old, traffic accident, longitudinal TB fracture on the right. Since then, hearing loss in right ear, tinnitus and unsteadiness. Examination: moderate sensorineural loss, steeply falling off in the high frequencies. Caloric excitability bilaterally equal, evoked nystagmus==>left. Surgery after 13 months: fine fissure across the tympanal region of the FN canal, running down to the OW. The fissure continued beyond the footplate toward the RW, without actually reaching it. The annular ligament was torn anteriorly to the fissure, with discharge of perilymph. RW intact. The fistula was covered by connective tissue. After surgery, the tinnitus and dizziness improved initially, but the dizziness reappeared after 10 more days.

4 months later, the right labyrinth could no longer be calorically excited. Surgical revision: intact mucous membrane over the anterior rim of the footplate with a perilymph pocket underneath. The mucous membrane was elevated and the defect once more closed with connective tissue. No improvement of hearing or lessening of the dizziness after 4 additional months.

Case 2. Male, 7 years old. Right TM perforated by a Q tip; vertigo and spontaneous nystagmus==>left. Examination: mixed-type hearing loss right, especially in the high frequencies. Surgery after 24 h: TM ruptured in posterosuperior quadrant; ossicular chain intact, but stapes luxated into vestibule; discharge of perilymph at the anterior margin of the footplate. The stapes could be repositioned, but did not stay in position. Footplate was left 1 or 2 mm under its normal level; fistula covered with connective tissue. After 3 months, neither dizziness, nor nystagmus; hearing normal.

Case 3. Male, 59 years old. Femur broken in an accident; general anesthesia to reposition it by means of a pin; afterwards, hearing loss right. Hearing improved spontaneously within 2 weeks. Following another general anesthesia, renewed hearing loss right and tinnitus. Examination: severe sensorineural hearing loss; nystagmus on left gaze; caloric excitability bilaterally equal. Ear surgery 4 months after first anesthesia accident: annular ligament torn on side facing the promontory and rupture of the RW membrane at its posterior rim; perilymphatic discharge from both windows; after their exposure, both defects were covered with connective tissue.

2 months later, hearing unchanged, tinnitus improved, no dizziness or nystagmus, caloric excitability bilaterally symmetrical.

In cases 1 and 2, an OW fistula existed, in case 3, combined lesions of both windows. The cause of the fistula in case 1 was a fissure running across the labyrinthine wall, continuing onto the annular ligament. In case 2, the stapes was depressed by a mechanical force acting via the EEC. In case 3, one must assume that the accident ruptured both windows, that both of them had healed spontaneously, but were ruptured again by some minor accident during the anesthesia: a rise in blood pressure, an alteration in the concentration of blood gases [52] or an increase in intracranial pressure caused by pressing or retching.

In the following 12 cases, the RW alone was ruptured:

Case 4. Female, 21 years old. Cholesteatoma on the left; emergency surgery because of a purulent meningitis; exact presurgical findings could not be established. When the cholesteatoma matrix was taken off the promontory, clear fluid surged from the RW niche. A window membrane was not found. The perilymph flow could only be controlled by pressing a large piece of connective tissue into the RW niche and packing the hypotympanum with gelfoam.

1 month postoperatively, moderate sensory hearing loss left, combined with a conductive loss of 45 dB. After 1 year, the cholesteatoma had recurred. The ear was deaf, but there was no vertigo. Surgical revision uncovered again a cholesteatoma, originating from the hypotympanum; it had eroded the promontory, exposed the basal turn and partly destroyed it. On removal of the cholesteatoma matrix, the perilymphatic space was once more opened but, this time, there was no surge of perilymph. After the defect in the labyrinthine wall had been covered by connective tissue, healing progressed without further incidents. The ear remained deaf, but there was no vertigo anymore.

Case 5. Female, 55 years old. Right ear deaf, immediately after cholesteatoma surgery; vertigo, first decreasing, then becoming stronger again. Spontaneous nystagmus==>left; right ear calorically unexcitable. Surgical revision after 7 months: the OW appeared normal; the RW was deeply recessed; perilymphatic discharge not clearly established. The niche to the RW was closed with connective tissue. Afterwards, the vertigo lessened, the nystagmus==>left persisted.

Case 6. Female, 37 years old. Left ear deaf, following ME surgery for chronic purulent otitis media. A surgical revision 6 months later did not uncover any cause for the deafness. 1 year postoperatively, dizzy spells and tinnitus. Examination: left ear completely deaf, no nystagmus, caloric excitability bilaterally symmetrical. Surgical exploration of the ME 4 years after the original operation: normal footplate; RW membrane only partly visible, no perilymphatic discharge. Because a fistula was suspected, the RW niche was closed with connective tissue. Postsurgically, ear remained deaf but, during the past 3 years, there was no recurrence of vertigo or tinnitus.

Common to cases 4–6 is the fact that the RW had been ruptured in connection with an otitis media or during surgery for an otitis. In case 4, the window membrane was apparently destroyed by the cholesteatoma. Whether or not the disease process had extended into the labyrinth at the time of the first surgery cannot be stated with certainty, since patient could not be examined beforehand. Postsurgically hearing was good. The gusher phenomenon indicated that the cochlear aqueduct was widely patent, an observation that could possibly be in contrast to the assertion by *Palva and Dammert* [337], who believed that, in the presence of an infection (meningitis or labyrinthitis), the aqueduct should be closed by swollen soft tissues. At the occasion of the surgical revision 1 year later, however, there was no recurrence of the perilymphatic upwelling; obviously, the patency of the aqueduct had changed in the interim. How the window rupture was brought about in the 2 other cases is not clear, since the surgical reports definitely indicated that the RW membrane was never touched. It is quite possible however that the membrane had been damaged by the preceding ME infection [251, 419].

Case 7. Male, 7 years old. Moderate sensorineural hearing loss left and severe deafness right; both had existed for some time. Approximately 1 h after a fall from a swing, the left ear became completely deaf. Examination: only residual hearing on left; no nystagmus, caloric excitability bilaterally equal. Infusion therapy without any success. 3 weeks after the accident, the left ME was opened surgically: the RW membrane was completely absent; window closed with pieces of connective tissue. Postsurgically, no improvement of hearing after 2 months.

Case 8. Male, 64 years old. When awakening in the morning, experienced hearing loss right and tinnitus; vertigo a few hours later. Examination: right ear deaf. Evoked nystagmus ==> left, positional nystagmus while lying on the left side. Right ear calorically hypoexcitable. Infusion therapy without effect. Surgery on the 11th day: large central defect in the RW membrane; closed over by connective tissue. Deafness persisted postsurgically; but there was no longer any tinnitus; vertigo considerably improved. After 6 months, no nystagmus, but right ear still calorically hypoexcitable.

Case 9. Male, 58 years old. While tearing out a bush in the garden, noticed sudden hearing loss left. Examination: severe mixed hearing loss left ear, increasing toward the high frequencies. During infusion therapy, vertigo and spontaneous nystagmus==>right. Otoscopically, fluid level behind left TM. Surgery 5 days later: blood coagulum in the RW niche, clear fluid underneath; fistula opening not visible. Vertigo subsided postsurgically; no nystagmus after 5 months; caloric excitability bilaterally equal. After 6 months, hearing normal in left ear, except for a 4-kHz notch of 40 dB.

Case 10. Male, 17 years of age. After a blow to the head, tinnitus in left ear; 1 h later, vertigo and vomiting. Examination: left ear completely deaf; spontaneous nystagmus==>right; fluid level behind TM. Surgery on same day: tear in the middle of the RW membrane, strong perilymphatic discharge. Niche packed with connective-tissue pieces. Vertigo and nystagmus subsided within 6 days; hearing normal after 6 weeks, only slight tinnitus remaining.

In patients 7–10, the RW had either been ruptured after a minor trauma (cases 7, 10), on increased intrathoracic pressure (case 9) or without a recognizable cause (case 8). Assuming preexisting weaknesses of the RW membranes, one might list these cases under *Althaus'* [6] label of 'spontaneous perilymphatic fistulae'. Notice the strong perilymphatic discharge in patients 9 and 10, indicating widely patent cochlear aqueducts.

Case 11. Male, 3 years old. While playing, pushed a fine rod through the TM. A few hours later, vertigo and vomiting. Audiological and vestibular tests could not be conducted because patient did not cooperate. Surgery on the following day: TM rupture in the posteroinferior quadrant; RW membrane freely visible, lying directly in the projection of the TM perforation; there was a central RW perforation. When the stapes was touched, perilymph was discharged from the perforation; the latter was closed by connective tissue. Postsurgically, no more vertigo; normal hearing after 4 days.

Case 12. Male, 12 years of age. 2 weeks after a skull-brain trauma, neurosurgical intervention because of a frontobasal CSF leak. Thereafter, hearing loss right and vertigo. Examination: complete deafness on the right. Exploratory tympanotomy 4 weeks after the accident: OW normal; subtotal defect of the RW membrane with discharge of perilymph; closed over with pieces of connective tissue. 4 weeks postsurgically, no vertigo, no nystagmus; after 3 months, ear continued to be deaf.

Case 13. Male, 21 years old. Following a car accident, hearing loss and tinnitus left. Examination: severe sensorineural hearing loss left; rotatory positional nystagmus==>left, when lying on the left side; caloric excitability equal on both sides. Surgery after 8 days: no defect in, or discharge of perilymph from, either window. In spite of that, RW niche packed with connective-tissue pieces. After 10 weeks, tinnitus lessened, hearing improved by 30 dB over the entire frequency range.

In cases 11–13, traumata had occurred, sufficiently strong to account for the RW lesions (case 11: transmeatal trauma; cases 12 and 13: blunt head trauma). With respect to case 12, one question remains open: Did the original trauma and the general anesthesia together produce the window rupture, similar to the situation in case 3? The endocranial surgery might have constituted an additional complicating factor.

Case 14. Male, 40 years old. After a brain concussion 26 years earlier, experienced dizziness and vomiting for the first time. Following a trivial head trauma 2 years later, renewed dizzy spells. Examination at that time revealed a low-frequency conductive hearing loss on the right, no nystagmus, caloric excitability equal on both sides. Continuing dizzy spells during the next 6 months; diagnosed as Menière's disease. No further complaints until about 1 year ago. Since then, hearing loss progressing on the right and tinnitus, sensation of fullness in the ear and dizzy spells. Examination: flat hearing loss right, somewhat worse in the low frequencies. No loss for speech discrimination; slight evoked nystagmus==>left; right ear calorically somewhat hypoexcitable. Negative glycerol test. Contrast filling of the right inner meatus gave ambiguous results. Surgical exploration of the right ME; complaint of vertigo when suction tube was accidentally applied to hypotympanum, minute perforation in the scarred RW membrane; closed over by connective tissue. After 3 weeks, dizziness lessened, hearing unchanged.

Case 15. Male, 59 years of age. Skull-base fracture 20 years earlier. Since then, hearing loss left and dizziness, i.e. a continual sensation of falling backwards. 2 years ago, brain concussion. Thereafter vertigo, especially on head turning. Examination: severe sensorineural hearing loss, increasing toward high frequencies; evoked nystagmus==>right; left ear calorically hypoexcitable. Findings at surgery: longitudinal fracture of the posterior wall of the EEC, incus subluxated, defect in the RW membrane; closed over by connective tissue. Time too early for evaluation of postsurgical results.

In patients 14 and 15, symptoms appeared a long time after a head trauma. Subsiding initially, they reappeared after an additional, trivial trauma (case 15) or without any recognizable cause (case 14). In the latter case, the course of events, together with the findings of a scarred window membrane at surgery, suggest that the RW had spontaneously healed after having been ruptured at the occasion of the first trauma. The scar was apparently not strong enough so that it was torn again later on. This patient could have been easily mistaken for a case of Menière's disease if it had not been for the negative glycerol test, a result which is in contrast to earlier findings [12] described in chapter 7.2.

7.5.2. Discussion of Case Reports

Considering these cases as a whole, one cannot recognize any preference of the trauma for one given side or for a certain age bracket. Women were less frequently involved than men (ratio 4:11), a tendency that had been found to exist also with respect to other forms of ear injuries. Ruptures of the RW membrane (12 cases) were more frequently found than isolated lesions of the annular ligament (2 cases) and combined injuries of both windows (1 case). This is different from what had to be expected from the literature. The various causes are once more listed in table LXXVIII.

OW fistulae were invariably located at the anterior rim of the footplate. Some RW perforations were central, others were marginal. In several cases, the site of the lesion could not be demonstrated, even though the mucous membrane folds and the promonotry lip had been removed.

The signs and symptoms varied. Hearing losses existed in all cases. 11 patients complained of dizziness (73%), 7 of tinnitus (47%). (In these respects, cases 4 and 9 must be disregarded, since presurgical audiometric examinations could not be conducted.) Uniform signs and symptoms

Table LXXVIII. Causes of window lesions in the Tübingen patients

Chronic middle ear infection	3
Blunt skull trauma	3
Skull trauma and temporal bone fracture	2
Accident and subsequent general anesthesia	2
Transmeatal injury	2
Blast trauma	1
Increased intrathoracic pressure	1
Unknowns ('spontaneous')	1
Total	15

characteristic of perilymphatic fistulae could not be established on the basis of the present patient material. Of the 13 ears with demonstrated hearing losses, 6 were completely deaf, 2 had severe flat hearing losses, 2 others severe high-frequency hearing losses, 1 a moderate hearing loss, increasing toward high frequencies, 1 other a moderate progressive hearing loss, especially in the low frequencies, and 1 more a mixed hearing loss. 1 patient with a moderate hearing loss did not show a loss for speech discrimination, an observation that is in contrast to the findings of other authors [109, 184, 273].

The vestibular signs and symptoms varied in a similar manner: 11 patients complained of dizziness. Of these, 1 patient (case 11) could not be examined before surgery. Of the remaining 10, 1 patient showed spontaneous nystagmus toward the involved ear, 4 spontaneous nystagmus toward the uninvolved ear, 3 an evoked nystagmus toward the uninvolved ear and 1 a positional nystagmus when lying on the side of the *uninvolved* ear. Positional nystagmus when patient is lying on the side of the *involved* ear is said to be characteristic of fistulae [109, 141, 183]. This was seen only once, and that in a patient who did not complain of dizziness at all (case 13). A gaze nystagmus when patient was looking toward the side of the uninvolved ear was also seen once, again in a patient who did not complain about dizziness (case 3). In only 8 of the 11 patients suffering from dizziness could caloric tests be conducted. In 5 of them, the involved ear was hypoexcitable or nonexcitable; in the 3 others, excitability was bilaterally equal.

In 1 patient (case 1), the fistula recurred after surgery. In all other, it had apparently been closed. Table LXXIX does not include case 4, since his presurgical auditory and vestibular functions were not known. Case 15 was also excluded, since the postsurgical results are not yet available, whereas case 11, who had regained normal hearing after surgery, was included.

By and large, the functional results agreed rather well with those cited in

Table LXXIX. Perilymphatic fistulae: functional results after surgical closure (percentages given in parentheses)

Symptom	Return to normal	Improved	Unchanged
Hearing loss	4	1	8
(n = 13)	(31)	(8)	(61)
Vertigo	6	3	1
(n = 10)	(60)	(30)	(10)
Tinnitus	2	4	–
(n = 6)	(33)	(67)	

the literature survey of chapter 7.3 — inasmuch as can be expected considering the present small number of cases. All patients in whom hearing returned to normal after surgery had been operated early: on the day of the
accident (case 10), on the next day (cases 2 and 11), on the fifth day (case 9).
(One may even include patient 13 in this list; he was operated on the 13th
day and had shown a moderate improvement.) The 3 patients operated after
longer time intervals (case 8 on the 11th day, case 12 on the 14th and case
7 on the 21st day) remained completely deaf after surgery, and so did the
other patients who were not operated until after even longer time intervals,
months or even years.

7.6. Our Postmortem Findings

The method for preparing the human TB, obtained from patients who
had died directly following a skull trauma, was described in chapter 2.2.
Even though the RW was approached from the hypotympanum, thus permitting the best possible view into the niche, a complete exposure of the
window membrane was not feasible until all mucous membrane folds had
been removed and the promontory lip taken down.

The following pathological findings were made on the RW and its immediate environment:

In 2 specimens, the RW membrane was destroyed during the removal of
the TB. Hence, their status could not be assessed. The remaining 87 RW
membranes were evaluated.

In 3 cases, the RW niche was filled with scar tissue. After its removal,
the membranes were intact and appeared normal. In 2 of these 3 ears,
radical mastoidectomies had been carried out previously.

In 5 instances, the RW membrane was intact, although altered by scars.
In 1 case, strands of scar tissue ran toward the mucous membrane folds lying
farther laterally in the niche. Since death had occurred at or immediately
after the head trauma, these must have been old scars produced by earlier
traumata.

On the other hand, submucosal hemorrhages found in RW membranes
that were still intact should have been produced by the same trauma that
had caused patient's death. Such hemorrhages were found in 5 specimens:
following serious head injuries with fractures of the cranial vault; after grave
soft-tissue injuries without bone fractures, and after a gunshot injury.

In 2 instances, the RW membrane was not injured, but its osseous rim was split, in 1 case, by a fissure running across the promontory from the OW to the RW (gunshot injury with a homolateral, longitudinal TB fracture), in the other, by a fine fissure originating at the RW and terminating somewhere around the subiculum (concurrent homolateral fracture of the cranial vault, no TB fracture).

In 1 other specimen, the entire labyrinth, including the osseous frame of the RW, was split in two by a lateral transversal fracture. The window membrane was torn. The frame of the OW was fractured along its short axis and the footplate in its anterior portion.

Torn RW membranes, without concomitant fractures of their osseous frames, were found in 5 cases. 1 of them was a simple, radially running slit (accompanying a fracture of the cranial vault), another one a double slit, also running radially (concurrent with a brain concussion); in neither case was a fracture of the TB present. In the third case, the RW membrane was torn off from the caudal rim of the niche (in the presence of a TB fracture). In the fourth case, there was a subtotal defect of the membrane; only a small margin remained posteriorly (accompanying a fracture of the cranial vault that had not involved the TB). In the fifth case, there was a minute, roundish, central perforation in a window membrane that showed older scars and was retracted (simultaneous fracture of the homolateral squama, no fracture of the TB proper). In the last case, the membrane had evidently been altered by scars. In the first 3 cases, the membranes did not show any scars. In the fourth case, the original condition of the membrane could no longer be judged.

With the exception of the case with the transversal fracture just mentioned, injuries to the footplate or to the annular ligament were not observed.

To summarize at this point, it may be stated that, among the 87 TB examined, 13 showed definite signs of injury to the RW membrane or its immediate environment (15%). In 5 of them (6% of the total), there was nothing but a rupture of the window membrane (table LXXX).

Table LXXX. Round window findings in 87 temporal bone specimens

Intact, normal appearance	69
Intact, scarred	5
Intact, fissure in osseous rim	2
Subepithelial hematoma	5
Ruptured (membrane only)	5
Ruptured (labyrinthine fracture)	1

7.7. Our Animal Experiments

Animal experiments were conducted in an effort to study the self-repair of the RW membrane. In particular, the experiments were designed to find out if this repair might be influenced by the mode of injury, e.g. by increases in intracranial pressure in accordance with the so-called 'explosive' mode of window rupture [144, 175, 303].

7.7.1. Material and Methods

In 28 guinea pigs, the tympanic bulla was opened under Nembutal anesthesia. Only healthy appearing animals were utilized. Nevertheless, in 3 animals an otitis media was detected during surgery. All 3 of them were retained in the experimental series. The RW membrane was lanced in its central section with a 17-gauge needle, producing a small slit that extended over about two thirds of its diameter. In 18 animals, the perforation in 1 ear was made in the manner just described, i.e. mechanically, in the other with a thermocautery needle. Pieces of gelfoam soaked with Tetracyclin were put into the bulla of 20 animals before the soft tissues were closed by sutures. In 7 animals, the dura of the posterior fossa was exposed by drilling away the occipital squama. The defect was merely closed over by skin. This soft spot later on facilitated compression of the subdural space by a finger in order to increase the CSF pressure [2]. In this manner, transient pressure increases were produced twice daily for 3 min each in the animals thus operated. By letting the head dangle or by compressing the thorax [303] attempts were made to raise the intracranial pressure even further.

After surviving for 1-6 weeks, the animals were sacrificed. The TB were removed and decalcified in an ethylenediaminetetraacetic acid (EDTA) solution. The specimens were then cut and the individual slides stained with HE or trichromic acid.

7.7.2. Results

In 44 specimens it was possible to evaluate the condition of the RW membrane under the light microscope. In 4 cases, a perforation was still present; the free rims carried small pads (fig. 11). or were beset by granulation tissue. In 11 cases, the membrane had healed completely; its three layers were easily recognized and there were no signs of scars (fig. 12). In 5 specimens, the membrane was thickened in a narrow area, presumably the region of the healed perforation. In 2 cases, there was a double membrane, as if the wound margins growing out from either side had not precisely met each other, but had simply reached the opposite osseous rim on their own. 9 membranes were intact, but showed granulation tissue in circumscribed areas either on their bullar side (7 membranes), on their cochlear side (1 membrane) or on both sides (1 membrane) (fig. 13). In 5 other cases, these granulations were so abundant that they filled the entire window area. Fibrous strands could be recognized running radially, i.e. in the direction of the

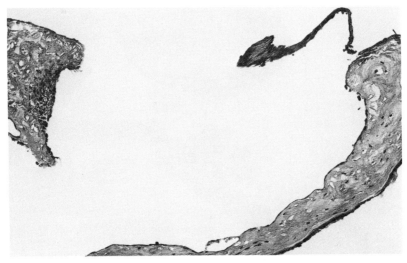

Fig. 11. Experimentally produced round window defect (guinea pig), 7 days after mechanical injury. Note the small pad on the free rim of the perforation. HE. × 125.

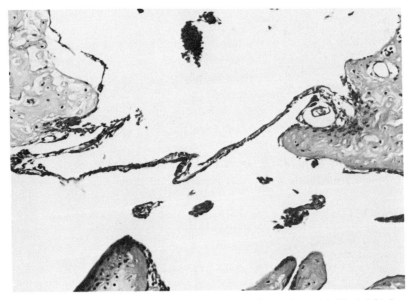

Fig. 12. Experimentally produced round window defect (guinea pig). Healed 21 days after mechanical injury. No visible scar. The fold was produced during preparation. HE. × 125.

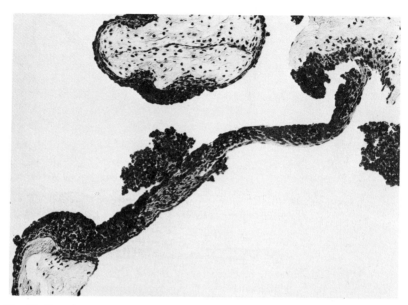

Fig. 13. Experimentally produced round window defect (guinea pig). Membrane 21 days after thermal injury, intact; swollen membrana propria; polypoid granulation tissue on the tympanal surface. Trichrom. × 125.

normal fiber structure of the membrane, but there was no epithelial stratum (fig. 14). In 4 specimens, the RW was closed over by loose granulation tissue or by connective tissue in which no fibers could be recognized. In the 4 last specimens, there was newly formed bone behind a window that was partly membraneous and partly replaced by connective tissue. This bone sealed the basal turn almost completely off from the RW. Table LXXXI summarizes these findings.

In 20 ears, there was an otitis media, in some of them of the serous type, in others granulation tissue was present. 2 of these infections had already

Table LXXXI. Experimental round window perforation: findings in 44 guinea pigs

Persisting perforation	4
Intact and transparent	11
Intact, but thickened (double membrane in two instances)	7
Intact with circumscribed small granulations	9
Window filled with granulation tissue	5
Window filled with connective tissue, no membrane structure present	4
Newly formed bone behind the window	4

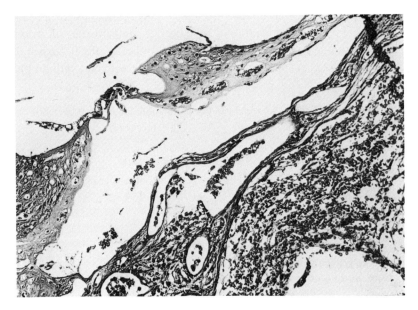

Fig. 14. Experimentally produced round window defect (guinea pig). 35 days after thermal injury. Window filled with loose connective tissue; membrane fibers running in normal directions. The cochlea is protected, no labyrinthitis present. HE. × 125.

existed before surgery. In 1 of the latter animals, histology revealed microabscesses in the mucous membrane. A third otitis media that had also been seen during surgery had completely cleared up after 3 weeks.

A labyrinthitis was found in 15 ears. There was proliferation of loose connective tissue in the basal turn of scala tympani, less frequently in the higher turns. (Counted among these 15 ears are the 4 with osteogenesis in scala tympani.) In 12 of the 15, there was also an otitis media. However, in 3 of these ears bulla and ME were entirely free of infection.

Table LXXXII correlates the histological findings with the two modes of RW injury employed. When the injury was produced by cautery, healing was apparently not worse than when it was produced mechanically, especially since all persisting perforations found had occurred after mechanical injuries. The only difference encountered between the two types of injury concerned the occurrence of granulation tissue on the membrane. After cautery, it was found twice as frequently as after mechanical injury. The same difference existed with respect to otitis media. It is conceivable therefore that the heat trauma predisposes the ME mucosa to inflammatory reactions.

A second factor that might have affected the results was the elevation of intracranial pressure, which should have been accompanied by an increase in intralabyrinthine pressure. As table LXXXIII indicates, the incidence of successful window repair was approximately the same with and without pressure

Table LXXXII. Experimental round window perforation: the effect of the mode of injury (percentages given in parentheses)

	Perforation made	
	mechanically (n = 31)	thermally (n = 13)
Persisting perforation	4 (13)	–
Intact and transparent	8 (26)	3 (23)
Intact and thickened	6 (19)	1 (8)
Intact with granulations	5 (16)	4 (31)
Window filled with granulation tissue	3 (10)	2 (15)
Window filled with connective tissue, no membrane structure present	3 (10)	1 (8)
Newly formed bone behind the window	2 (6)	2 (15)
Otitis media	12 (39)	8 (61)
Labyrinthitis	10 (32)	5 (38)

Table LXXXIII. Experimental round window perforation: the effect of periodically increased perilymphatic pressure (percentages in parentheses)

	No pressure increase (n = 32)	Periodic pressure increases (n = 12)
Persisting perforation	3 (9)	1 (8)
Intact and transparent	7 (22)	4 (34)
Intact and thickened	4 (12.5)	3 (25) (double membranes in 2 cases)
Intact with granulations	6 (19)	2 (25)
Window filled with granulation tissue	4 (12.5)	1 (8)
Window filled with connective tissue, no membrane structure present	4 (12.5)	–
Newly formed bone behind the window	4 (12.5)	–
Otitis media	16 (50)	4 (33)
Labyrinthitis	13 (41)	2 (17)

increases. There was one possible exception. Both ears in which the double RW membranes were found belonged in the group that was repeatedly exposed to pressure increases. Hence, transient increases in perilymphatic pressure could possibly prevent the wound margins from lining up properly with each other, although it might not hinder their primary tendency to proliferate.

Labyrinthitis was much less frequently seen in the group that was exposed to repeated pressure increases. However, in view of the small number of cases, this could well be an accidental finding. If confirmed, however, it would suggest that the frequently induced perilymphatic discharges via the perforated window membrane might, to some extent, minimize the chances of germs to enter the labyrinth.

The study facilitated the examination of two side issues: (a) the effect of prophylactive topical application of antibiotics on the occurrence of postsurgical otitis media and/or labyrinthitis, and (b) the influence of both kinds of infection on the self-repair of the RW membrane (tables LXXXIV, LXXXV).

Table LXXXIV. Experimental round window perforation: the effect of prophylactive topical antibiotics

	Antibiotics (n = 28)	No antibiotics (n = 16)
Otitis media present/absent	13/15	7/9
Labyrinthitis present/absent	8/20	7/9
Persisting perforation present/absent	2/26	2/14

Table LXXXV. Experimental round window perforation: the influence of otitis media and/or labyrinthitis

	Otitis media present/absent	Labyrinthitis present/absent
Total	20/24	15/29
Persisting perforation	0/4	0/4
Intact and transparent	1/10	0/11
Intact and thickened	4/3	0/7
Intact with granulations	5/4	3/6
Window filled with granulation tissue	4/1	4/1
Window filled with connective tissue, no membrane structure present	4/0	4/0
Newly formed bone behind the window	2/2	4/0

In 1 case, the otitis media that existed before surgery healed, perhaps under the influence of the antibiotics given. It persisted in the 2 other cases, in which it had also been present before surgery, but where no antibiotics were given. However, in general topical antibiotics do not seem to have influenced the ratio of postoperative otitis media. On the other hand, labyrinthitis occurred at a much lesser rate under prophylactic antibiotic treatment than without it. Thus, the efficacy of topical antibiotics could not be determined with certainty on the basis of the present experiments.

Properly healed RW membranes — but also persisting perforations — were almost exclusively found in ears free of otitis media. Membranes beset with granulations were more frequently seen when there was an otitis. When there was a combination of otitis media and labyrinthitis, changes of the RW membrane were especially severe with formation of granulations and intracochlear growth of connective tissue. Deposition of bone behind the RW was found only when a labyrinthitis was present.

One additional factor affecting the membrane repair might be the time of observation after surgery. Several animals died between the weekly intevals planned for their sacrifice. Therefore, the time distribution listed in table LXXXVI occasionally deviated from strict weekly intervals.

Table LXXXVI. Experimental round window perforation: the effect of the time of sacrifice

	Time of sacrifice (days after injury)							
	1	7–9	12–14	21	28	35	42	Total number in each row
Persisting perforation	1	3						4
Intact and transparent		3	2	3	2	1		11
Intact and thickened		1*		3*	2	1		7
Intact with granulations			3	2	2	1	1	9
Window filled with granulation tissue		2		1		2		5
Window filled with connective tissue, no membrane structure present			1		3			4
Newly formed bone behind the window				1	1		2	4
Total number in each column	1	9	6	10	10	5	3	44

* Double membrane

Table LXXXVI indicates that all persisting perforations were found during the first 9 days. Nevertheless, 6 other membranes had completely healed during the same time period. Severe forms of changes, such as loss of the membrane structure and osteogenesis within the cochlea, were only seen after longer time intervals. All other findings were fairly evenly distributed over the time of observation.

Finally, the impression was gained that the condition of the RW membrane, as well as that of the basal turn of scala tympani behind it, were, as a rule, similar in the 2 ears of a given animal, even though the mode of injury differed. All but 6 of the 16 animals, in which both ears could be evaluated, showed essentially similar findings in both ears. It may be worth noting that there was not a single case in the entire series with bilaterally persisting perforations.

7.7.3. Discussion of Animal Experiments

Chances for self-repair of RW membranes appear quite good. Of the 44 ears with experimental ruptures that could be evaluated, only 4 showed persisting perforations, but none later than the ninth day. Apparently, the mode of injury, mechanical or thermal, did not noticeably affect the repair. Periodic elevations of the intracranial pressure were also without an effect, except possibly in the 2 animals in which the wound margins did not exactly meet. Although proliferating properly, they stayed at different levels, producing a dual membrane. It is quite conceivable that the repeated perilymphatic discharges provoked by the pressure elevations were responsible for this defective repair. On the other hand, the same discharges might have prevented the entry of infectious agents and thus the development of a labyrinthitis.

Neither otitis media nor labyrinthitis did completely prevent the repair of the RW membrane. However, they promoted the growth of granulation tissue on its surface (otitis media) or contributed to the dissolution of its structure (labyrinthitis). Hence, injuries of the RW membrane may invite inflammatory reactions of the inner ear, and these in turn may lead to structural changes in the window region. These results are in good agreement with histological findings on *human* temporal bones [46, 419]. In 1 case of an RW rupture [46], connective-tissue proliferation had been seen in the basal cochlear turn. In the other, a fracture of the labyrinth and rupture of the RW [419], new bone had formed behind it; furthermore, the free rim of the perforation had been thickened into a small pad, in exactly the same manner as was found in our own animal experiments (cf. fig. 11).

As already stated, all 4 persisting perforations of the current series were observed within a time period of not more than 9 days after the injury. After longer time intervals, the RW had invariably healed. This agrees quite well with the findings of *Axelsson* et al. [16], who saw only one perforation persisting beyond the tenth day in a series of 13 animals. Therefore, the healing of RW ruptures appears to be mainly a matter of time. On the other hand, it is quite possible that constitutional factors might also affect both the capability of the RW to repair itself and the reactions of the inner ear to the injury. This notion could perhaps be supported by the fact that findings were frequently bilaterally symmetrical. (However, in guinea pigs, otitis media, if present, almost invariably exist in both ears, possibly because of their relatively wide Eustachian tubes [435].)

7.8. Discussion of Round Window Injuries and Perilymphatic Fistulae

The notion of *Goodhill* [144], to separate RW membrane ruptures into those caused by 'explosive' pulses and others caused by 'implosive' pulses, is attractive at first sight because of its simplicity. However, it can neither be supported by the numerous observations reported in the literature nor by our own findings.

As may be recalled, *Goodhill* [144] assumed that intracranial pressure pulses should be transmitted into the perilymphatic space via the cochlear aqueduct and/or along the cochlear nerve fibers. In this manner, they would displace the windows or, in extreme cases, rupture them ('explosive' pulses). In a reverse manner, sudden pressure increases in the ME (Valsalva maneuver) or in the EEC should displace the stapes into the vestibule and, consequently, the RW membrane into scala tympani ('implosive' pulses).

The existence of a communication between the CSF space and the perilymphatic space can no longer be denied neither for the case of experimental (mammalian) animals nor for that of humans. (For details cf. chapter 7.4.) It appears, however, that this communication is widely patent only in a few human subjects, as is indicated by the relatively rare finding of a gusher [185, 309]. Neither roentgenological nor histological studies were successful so far in demonstrating the cause(s) of such abnormal patencies. Moreover, case 4 of chapter 7.5.1 showed that a gusher encountered during a first surgical intervention was found drastically reduced in strength within one year at the occasion of a second intervention. Apparently, it is not simply the lumen of the osseous canal as such, but alterations of its soft-tissue lining, not yet understood, that determine the variable patency of the cochlear aqueduct (and possibly also that of the spiral tractus foraminosus). *Palva and Dammert* [337] as well as *Waltner* [454] had entertained similar notions, although the role played in this connection by the barrier membrane of *Waltner*'s is still unresolved.

There are some general, purely physical reasons that argue strongly against *Goodhill*'s [144] above-mentioned concept. In general, narrow channels, like the aqueduct (not to mention the openings of the spiral tractus foraminosus), provide frictional damping, the more so the longer and narrower they are. Such channels act as *low-pass* filters. This means (a) that pulses are attenuated on transmission, and (b) that they are delayed in time and extended in duration: they are being *'smeared out in time'*. An audible pulse, for example, changes from a sharp crack to a dull thud under such a condition [435].

With respect to the aqueduct, this general principle was confirmed by the observations of *Kobrak* [253] and *Myers* [323] that were already mentioned: a rise in intracranial pressure was transmitted into the perilymphatic space, but it became attenuated and was delayed in time. Hence, the notion that a CSF pressure pulse generated by a head trauma could rapidly and in full strength reach the RW membrane via the cochlear aqueduct is quite untenable.

Intracranial pressure increases that rise slowly but are maintained for longer time periods may well be capable of injuring or even rupturing the window membrane [2, 175, 303]. Such pressure elevations are brought about, for instance, when a person presses, when the blood pressure is raised [52] or during artificial respiration [136, 434]. (The steady-state portions of such quasi-stationary pressure changes are not affected by the above-mentioned low-pass filter restraint; only their onsets and terminations may be rendered more gradual.)

As regards the 'implosive' cause, the following comments are in order: an increased ME pressure primarily affects the TM because its surface is much larger than that of the 2 windows, alone or in combination. During a Valsalva maneuver, for instance, the net displacement of the stapes is in an *outward* direction and, during a pressure rise in the EEC, in an *inward* direction. That pressure rises in the EEC may actually be transmitted to the inner ear and elevate its pressure in turn was demonstrated by *Tjernström* [e.g. 493], although only for relatively small increments in EEC pressure.

Nevertheless, alterations of the environmental pressure may produce a pressure differential between the CSF space and the perilymphatic space on the one hand and the ME on the other, as long as there is no equilibration via the Eustachian tube. During diving, for example, the environmental pressure may rise rapidly. The excess pressure is transmitted to the fluid-filled spaces of the body, but not to the ME (again, only if the Eustachian tube fails to open), but it also acts on the TM and thus indirectly on the inner ear. If at this point the Valsalva maneuver is successfully executed, the pressure differential between the fluid spaces and the ME is lessened and the pressure acting on the TM (and thus on the inner ear) is also reduced. If the ME cannot be aerated — for example when the difference between the environmental pressure and that in the ME is in excess of 90 mm Hg [280] — the Valsalva maneuver, by increasing the intrathoracic pressure, may elevate the CSF and intralabyrinthine pressures even further and thus make the pressure differential between the fluid spaces and the ME still larger. Such a mechanism may indeed lead to a rupture of the RW membrane, an opinion that is shared by *Freeman* [132].

The above line of reasoning argues strongly against the notion of *Althaus* [6], i.e. that the RW membrane could be ruptured 'implosively' when the communication between the CSF space and the perilymphatic space is blocked. On the contrary, an open communication is one of the conditions needed to produce a pressure elevation behind the RW membrane in the manner just outlined.

Ruptures of the RW membrane were reported to have occurred on relatively small elevations of pressure in the EEC as well as within the thorax, such as produced by laughing, coughing, sneezing, etc. The mode of the trauma is essentially the same as that just described, only the order of magnitude of the underlying labyrinthine-pressure elevation is surprisingly small. Animal experiments [175, 303] revealed that the resistance of the RW membrane against its rupture varies widely, in a manner similar to that found for the case of the TM [473]. In addition, one must consider some other facts: (a) that scars were seen in the RW membrane in 6% of the TB specimens examined; (b) that ME infections might lead to a weakening of the RW membrane [251], and (c) that weak areas might exist on a congenital basis [5] which, by the way, were also demonstrated in the annular ligament [27]. It is therefore quite feasible that such a weakened membrane might be ruptured by an accidental trivial trauma. There should be a gradual transition between such an event and the rupture of a normal membrane by a higher pressure.

The transfer of quasi-stationary CSF pressure elevations via the cochlear aqueduct is certainly an important cause of elevations in perilymphatic pressure but, most likely, it is not the only one. *Carlborg* [52] found perilymphatic pressure elevations on changes in the partial pressures of blood gases. However, he did not examine the question whether such perilymphatic pressure elevations might be caused indirectly via changes in CSF pressure or by direct action on the labyrinth. Such changes, regardless of their source of origin, might play a role in RW membrane ruptures that occur in conjunction with a barotrauma.

It may be recalled that stemming the return flow of blood from the head, for example by the test of Queckenstedt or by an elevation in intrathoracic pressure, does not only aid in increasing the CSF pressure and the intralabyrinthine one [e.g. 323], but also in augmenting the blood volume in the inner-ear vessels and thus in elevating the intralabyrinthine pressure even further. As far as I am aware of, this potential cause of RW membrane ruptures has so far never been considered.

The mode of origin of RW ruptures that are produced by head trauma must still be clarified. A pressure pulse transmitted from the CSF space is definitely not the cause (cf. above). *Barnick* [20] as well as *Wittmaack* [467] already considered the possibility of transient deformations of the labyrinthine walls that might decrease the enclosed volume and thus increase the intralabyrinthine pressure. *Ulrich* [443] varied this notion slightly; he assumed that the deformation might produce a structural distortion of the osseous RW frame and thus of its membrane. The studies of *Guerrier* et al. [160] on the elastic deformation of the ME walls rendered this concept quite tenable.

Further support is found in the following observations of our own: (a) The fissures, found in some of the postmortem specimens, were located at the posterior aspect of the RW; or they ran across the promontory to the upper RW rim, or from the tympanal portion of the FN canal down toward the OW niche and onto the promontory, as in case 1 of chapter 7.5.1. (b) Lateral transversal fractures diagnosed either clinically or observed in the postmortem specimens, as a rule, ruptured both windows. Both of these findings suggest that, when the labyrinthine walls are being deformed during the course of a head trauma, the window region is the zone of the maximal bending moment. In a way similar to what has been demonstrated for the case of the cranial vault [452], transversal bending in this region should lead to osseous fractures or fissures and overstretching of the membranes to their rupture. Bulging of the footplate or the RW membrane caused by a rise in intralabyrinthine pressure may further aggravate such injuries.

The concepts underlying the terms 'explosive' and 'implosive' window ruptures [6, 144] were shown to be untenable. Yet, it is useful at times to indicate the direction of a given pressure differential. For that purpose, the terms 'excess internal pressure' and 'excess external pressure' are suggested. They include quasi-stationary pressure elevations and cover even instances, like case 10 of chapter 7.5.1, in which an excess external pressure was produced by a blow to the ear; its onset might have been rather sudden, but not quite explosive.

As was shown above, the two cochlear windows may be ruptured by excess internal or external pressures or by being overstretched when their frames are distorted. The extent of the resulting lesion will vary widely with the resistance of individual membranes. The following schema attempts to show the different modes of origin as well as the varying severity of the resulting trauma:

Excess internal pressure	*Overstretching*	*Excess external pressure*
Increased intra-thoracic pressure	Blunt skull trauma	Transmeatal trauma
Barotrauma		

↓   Trauma unnoticed ('spontaneous rupture')

Trivial trauma of a weakened membrane

Purely taumatic rupture of a normal membrane   ↓

Increasing membrane resistance   Severity of trauma

The notions of *Simmons* [399] and of *Goodhill* [144] about the effects of RW membrane ruptures on inner-ear structures and function are quite persuasive because of their cohesiveness but, again, they are incapable of accounting for all findings.

First of all, it is not immediately obvious why an increased pressure in the perilymphatic space should lead not only to the rupture of the RW membrane, but to the rupture of Reissner's membrane as well. *Simmons* [399] had stated that repairs of these two membranes should occur independently of each other so that the cochlear symptoms could subside while the perilymphatic fistula might still persist and vice versa. However, the cases he cited as evidence for his thesis rested on mere clinical impressions. A persisting RW fistula producing no signs and symptoms whatsoever was never demonstrated. On the other hand, when the fistula was surgically closed at an early stage, the auditory function frequently recovered and the dizziness became almost invariably less. These findings strongly suggest a cause-and-effect relation between the fistula and the impairments of inner-ear functions.

If the barrier membrane of *Waltner* [454] would rupture, CSF should enter the perilymphatic space and alter its electrolyte concentrations, but only as long as fluid is being discharged through the fistula. Repair of the endothelial structure could not be expected until the CSF flow has ceased; this would only happen when the RW membrane has healed.

It should finally be noted that in postmortem specimens both of experimental animals and of humans, examined after longer time intervals, parts of the cochlear spaces of varying sizes were found to be filled with fibrous or osseous tissue. However, it is not known if in such cases symptoms of a generalized labyrinthitis were ever observed earlier during life.

Signs and symptoms of ruptures of the cochlear windows vary widely. The characteristic triad, hearing loss, vertigo and tinnitus, is frequently observed, although patients displaying only one single symptom are by no means rare. The results of auditory as well as of vestibular tests range from completely normal to total functional deficits. None of the clinical test methods, such as the glycerol test and roentgenological examinations, provide unequivocal evidence for the presence of a perilymphatic fistula. The use of radioisotope markers in the CSF permits such a diagnosis if the results are positive, but does not negate it if the results are negative. Since this type of examination requires surgical exposure of the ME, it appears simpler, and more logical, to explore the tympanic cavity surgically and to inspect both windows directly when a fistula is suspected. In most cases, admittedly, the RW membrane cannot be seen in its entirety until the protruding osseous lip of the promontory and the mucous membrane folds within the niche have been removed. This was shown to be the case in our own postmortem examinations and also in the histological study of *Stewart and Belal* [419]. A mere endoscopic inspection of the ME cavity through a myringotomy opening, usually, does not provide sufficient information about the condition of the RW membrane, although the small intervention required would make it an attractive procedure.

At this point, some comments might be in order concerning the relation between perilymphatic fistulae and auditory impairment. The following theoretical considerations are submitted [435]: Drainage of perilymph upsets the normal pressure equilibrium between endolymph and perilymph with the result that cochlear sensitivity is reduced in a manner similar to what occurs during acute Menière attacks. If the drainage is intermittent, which is often the case, the pressure dysequilibrium should also be intermittent and the hearing loss should fluctuate. This mechanically induced loss should recover fully when the fistula is closed. However, the loss of perilymph may also affect the position of the endocochlear membranes and produce lesions by impairing the blood supply. (In contrast to Menière's disease, the pressure changes occur much more suddenly; thus, they are potentially more dangerous.) These effects will lead to a true sensory hearing loss that should not fluctuate, should even progress with time, and should not recover when the fistula is closed. There may be combinations of both forms so that the hearing loss partially recovers on closure of the fistula. Hence, losses that fluctuate should have a better prognosis than those that do not do so and gradually progress in severity, and early closure of the fistula should minimize permanent damage.

There are hardly any differences of opinion about the *management of RW ruptures*. Both the annular ligament and the RW membrane appear to repair themselves quite readily. Scars in the RW membrane are frequently found; other positive evidence is provided by clinical observations [60] as well as by findings in animal studies [16, 26, 400] (cf. also present chapter 7.7.2). Bed rest and avoidance of elevations in CSF pressure may aid the repair. Yet, occasional changes in CSF pressure do not appear to be particularly harmful, as was shown by our own animal experiments. Since the chances for maintaining auditory function, or for its recovery, decrease fast when the fistula remains open for some time, one should close it surgically as early as possible. Moreover, there is a good probability that the accompanying dizziness will also be lessened. The most suitable surgical approach appears to be to freshen the wound margins and to cover the opening with autologous connective tissue. Only a few recurrences have been described when this method was employed.

The audiometric results depend strongly on the time when the fistula is closed, as was indicated by the evaluation of the 80 cases reported in the literature and of the 15 observed in our own series. An additional advantage of early closure may lie in the fact that it would block a potential port of entry for germs and thus lessen the danger of a labyrinthitis.

8. General Summary

The effects of trauma on the middle ear, the potentials of various therapeutic measures employed and the results achieved were evaluated on a large series of patients seen at the Tübingen ENT Service over a period of 13 years. Furthermore, 89 postmortem specimens were examined; they had been obtained from persons who had died immediately following severe skull traumata. Finally, traumatic ruptures of the tympanic membrane and of the round window (RW) membrane were studied in animal experiments.

The monograph is divided into five parts: (1) injuries of the tympanic membrane (TM); (2) lesions of the ossicular chain; (3) endocranial complications of lesions of the middle ear (ME) and injuries of the facial nerve (FN); (4) cholesteatomata of traumatic origin, and (5) posttraumatic perilymphatic fistulae.

Evaluation of 531 *TM ruptures* aided in their analysis. The prevailing place of injury was the anteroinferior quadrant, regardless of the cause of injury, i.e. even when the TM had been ruptured in the course of blunt head traumata or in that of longitudinal fractures of the temporal bone (TB). Likewise, in the postmortem specimens, anteroinferior, central perforations were more frequently seen than posterosuperior, marginal perforations.

Explosions were found to produce TM injuries more frequently when the mastoid process showed little pneumatization. This finding is at variance with the concept generally accepted heretofore, i.e. that TM of ears with extensive pneumatization were more prone to injury, a notion that was based on a simplified interpretation of the physical gas laws. The pressure/volume characteristic of the TM as well as high-speed motion pictures taken while ruptures were occurring, together with theoretical considerations, suggested that the multiple-cell system of a highly pneumatized mastoid dampens the vibrations of the ME structures, protecting the TM of these ears to some degree against the effects of explosions.

Surgical adaptation of the wound margins and tympanoplastic procedures gave good results in 88% of patients, but only when carried out early, i.e. during the first week. When they were done during the second and third week, results became definitely poorer. Thereafter, up to the time of the third month, they became somewhat better once more, provided that tympanoplastic procedures were employed. A well-pneumatized mastoid aided the healing. After thermal injuries, surgical results turned out to be as good as after injuries of other causes. The chronological age of the patient did not influence the outcome. Audiometric results were the better the earlier the surgery was carried out. Following the second week after the trauma, they already became noticeably worse.

Analysis of *ossicular-chain lesions* was facilitated by the evaluation of 144 clinical patients and that of the 89 postmortem specimens. Luxation of the incus was the most frequent defect found (61%); fracture of the stapes was next in frequency (14%), whereas fractures and/or luxations of other parts of the chain or posttraumatic fixations were relatively rare (9%). The majority of these defects was caused by a blunt head trauma (75%), their incidence increasing with the severity of the trauma. Nevertheless, ossicular-chain lesions occurred also in the absence of laterobasal fractures and, quite frequently, even in the absence of TM injuries. In those cases, ossicular discontinuities might have been brought about by transient traumatic deformations of the TB, a notion suggested by experiments of other authors and supported by the present findings.

Straightforward instructions about the most suitable procedure for reconstructing an ossicular chain cannot be given. In general, the best functional results were obtained by the reposition of the ossicles and by the use of implants fashioned from stiff and biologically inert materials. The optimal time for this type of surgery was approximately 6 months after the original trauma.

Endocranial complications and FN injuries were assessed on 143 *laterobasal fractures*, observed in patients (122 longitudinal fractures, 17 transversal fractures and 4 with atypical courses), as well as in the 89 TB specimens. X-ray pictures, taken in the standard positions, provided correct diagnoses in 75% of the longitudinal fractures and in 57% of the transversal fractures.

The *endocranial complications* encountered included the following: 20 cases of cerebrospinal fluid (CSF) fistulae (of which 6 were surgically closed), 7 of otogenic meningitis (6 within the first 9 days after trauma, the 7th 16 years after a longitudinal fracture) and 2 cases of pneumatoceles. Dura lacerations healed quite well on their own so that they usually did not require surgical intervention. Those caused by lateral transversal fractures represented the exemption from this rule. Otogenic posttraumatic meningitis occurred most frequently in conjunction with highly shattered fractures and extensive soft tissue injuries in the ME. In these cases, the preventive surgical repair, originally recommended by *Voss* [450] is, in our opinion, still indicated.

The *FN* was injured in 88% of the transversal fractures and in 55% of the longitudinal ones. In clinical patients as well as in the postmortem specimens, the nerve was most frequently injured in the region of the geniculate ganglion (73% of cases). This finding contradicts the older rule, i.e. that the place of predilection would be the second knee. However, other sections of the FN were still so frequently involved that one cannot agree, without qualifications, with the opinion of *Fisch* [116], i.e. that the surgeon should always expose the geniculate ganglion directly via a transtemporal approach in every case of a posttraumatic FN palsy. In our experience, the safest surgical method lies in finding the fracture line first, wherever its location, then to trace it to the FN canal, expose the nerve and slit its sheath.

The prognosis of immediate palsies was not as good as that of early and late pareses (42% satisfactory results as compared to 60 or 63%, respectively). Decompression executed during the first week gave better results (good restoration of function in 73%) than waiting for spontaneous recovery. Although spontaneous recovery may still be expected as long as the nerve is electrically excitable, good functional results were obtained in only 61%.

The analysis of 22 patients with *posttraumatic cholesteatoma* revealed that it is brought about by a number of different modes of injury. The following is probably only a partial list: (a) keratinizing epithelium hemmed-in into a fracture cleft (99); (b) isolation of parts of the TM by bone fragments; (c) implantation of small pieces of epithelium into the ME; (d) inverted margins of ruptured TM, forming epithelial proliferations; (e) pockets within the TM that develop during its healing; (f) shattered fractures of the posterior wall of the EEC; (g) posttraumatic stenoses of the EEC, and (h) injuries to the Eustachian tube. ME cholesteatomata, formed late after trauma, were more frequently found than perusal of the contemporary literature suggests (6.1% in cases of fractures of the otobasis, 2.6% in cases of ruptured TM).

Injuries to the *RW membrane* were rarely recognized clinically (i.e. in only 13 patients), but their presence in 7% of the postmortem specimens suggests that they may quite frequently occur in conjunction with a blunt skull trauma. Most likely, they are caused by transient deformations of the labyrinthine walls, especially since the bending moment appears to be strongest in the region of the RW.

Consistent signs and symptoms characteristic of the rupture of the RW membrane could not be established. Hearing loss, almost invariably present, occurred in various forms and to varying degrees; dizziness (75% of all cases) and tinnitus (50%) were less constant. Surgical closure of the perforation usually lessened the dizziness and the tinnitus. Hearing was improved only when surgery was carried out early; the chances of improvement decreased exponentially with time after the trauma.

The animal experiments suggested that the capability of the RW membrane to repair itself is rather good: the membrane was experimentally perforated in 44 guinea pig ears. Merely 4 perforations were found to persist, and these only within the first 9 days. Nevertheless, a number of defective repairs were seen: double membranes, blockage of the window region by connective tissue scars, and osteogenesis in scala tympani. Experimental elevations of the CSF pressure did not affect the repair — with the possible exception of the formation of the double membranes, seen in 2 such cases.

The present study indicates that surgical exploration of the ME and, if required, its reconstruction, should be carried out early, whenever there are injuries to the TM, FN palsies, shattered fractures in the region of the ear (because of the danger of meningitis) and also when ruptures of the RW membrane are suspected. Only early surgery promises optimal results. *Uncomplicated* fractures of the otobasis are the exception. Surgery may be delayed, provided there are no serious complications that require immediate surgical intervention. Delaying surgery is especially indicated when an ossicular-chain lesion is suspected, as late reconstruction (i.e. after 6 months) provides better functional results than early surgery.

References

Part A

1 Agazzi, C.: Indications de la chirurgie pour lésions traumatiques des osselets. Acta oto-rhino-lar. belg. *25:*615–621 (1971).

2 Ahlén, G.: On the connection between cerebro-spinal and intralabyrinthine pressure and variations in the inner ear. Acta oto-lar. *35:*251–257 (1974).

3 Alexander, G.: Gesellschaftsbericht der österreichischen otologischen Gesellschaft. Zentbl. Ohrenheilk. *11:*190–192 (1913).

4 Allam, A.F.: Ruptur der Membran des runden Fensters. Z. Lar. Rhinol. *55:*544–548 (1976).

5 Althaus, S.R.: Spontaneous and traumatic perilymph fistulas. Laryngoscope, St Louis *87:*364–371 (1977).

6 Althaus, S.R.: Perilymph fistulas. Laryngoscope, St Louis *91:*538–562 (1981).

7 Altmann, F.; Basek, M.: Experimental fractures of the stapes in rabbits. Archs Otolar. *68:*173–193 (1958).

8 Andersen, H.C.; Elbrond, O.: Diagnose und Behandlung der isolierten Stapesfrakturen. Mschr. Ohrenheilk. *102:*87–90 (1968).

9 Andersen, H.C.; Jepsen, O.; Ratjen, E.: Ossicular chain defects. Diagnosis and treatment. Acta oto-lar. *54:*393–402 (1962).

10 Andreasson, L.; Ingelstedt, S.; Ivarsson, A.; Jonson, B.; Tjernström, Ö.: Pressure-dependent variation in volume of mucosal lining of the middle ear. Acta oto-lar. *81:*442–449 (1976).

11 Anson, B.J.; Donaldson, J.A.: Surgical anatomy of the temporal bone and ear (Saunders, Philadelphia 1973).

12 Arenberg, J.K.; May, M.; Stroud, M.H.: Perilymphatic fistula: an unusual cause of Menière's syndrome in a prepubertal child. Laryngoscope, St Louis *84:*243–246 (1974).

13 Armstrong, B.W.: Traumatic perforations of the tympanic membrane: observe or repair? Laryngoscope, St Louis *82:*1822–1830 (1972).

14 Arnold, W.; Ilberg, C. von: Neue Aspekte zur Morphologie und Funktion des runden Fensters. Z. Lar. Rhinol. *51:*390–399 (1972).

15 Arora, M.M.; Bhattacharya, T.; Mehra, Y.N.: Facial paralysis by direct transtympanal trauma. J. Laryng. *85:*983–984 (1971).

16 Axelsson, A.; Hallén, O.; Miller, J.M.; McPherson, D.L.: Experimentally induced round window membrane lesions. Acta oto-lar. *84:*1–11 (1977).

17 Azem, K.; Caldarelli, D.D.: Sudden conductive hearing loss following sneezing. Archs Otolar. *97:*413–414 (1973).

18 Ballance, C.; Duel, A.B.: The operative treatment of facial palsy by the introduction of

nerve grafts into the Fallopian canal by other intratemporal methods. Archs Otolar. *15*:1–70 (1932).

19 Ballantyne, J.: The surgical treatment of traumatic lesions of the auditory ossicles. Acta oto-rhino-lar. belg. *25*:622–640 1971).

20 Barnick, O.: Über Brüche des Schädelgrundes und die durch sie bedingten Blutungen in das Ohrlabyrinth. Arch. Ohrenheilk. *43*:23–52 (1897).

21 Bartlett, P.C.: Traumatic subluxation of the stapes. Ear Nose Throat J. *56*:214–216 (1977).

22 Bauer, F.: Dislocation of the incus due to head injury. J. Laryng. *72*:676–682 (1958).

23 Behbehani, A.; Kastenbauer, E.: Zur Ruptur und Läsion der Labyrinthfenster. Z. Lar. Rhinol. *57*:983–986 (1978).

24 Beickert, P.: Otosklerose (Otospongiose); in Berendes, Link, Zöllner, Hals-Nasen-Ohren-Heilkunde in Praxis und Klinik, Bd. V, 19.1–19.64 (Thieme, Stuttgart 1979).

25 Bellucci, R.J.; Fisher, E.G.; Rhodin, J.: Ultrastructure of the round window membrane. Laryngoscope, St Louis *82*:1021–1026 (1972).

26 Bellucci, R.J.; Wolff, D.: Repair and consequences of surgical trauma to the ossicles and oval window of experimental animals. Ann. Otol., St Louis *67*:400–429 (1958).

27 Bennett, R.J.: On subarachnoid-tympanic fistulae. A report of two cases of the rare indirect type. J. Laryng. *80*:1242–1252 (1966).

28 Berman, J.M.; Fredrickson, J.M.: Vertigo after head injury. A five-year follow-up. J. Otolaryngol. *7*:237–245 (1978).

29 Beselin, O.: Verbrennung des Mittelohres beim Eisenbrennen. HNO *4*:47 (1953).

30 Bezold, F.: Verbrühung des Trommelfells. Arch. Ohrenheilk. *18*:49–58 (1882).

31 Bezold, F.: Krankheiten des Warzenteiles; in Schwartze, Handbuch der Ohrenheilkunde, Bd. II, pp. 299–351 (Vogel, Leipzig, 1893).

32 Bichler, E.: Posttraumatische aseptische Nekrose des Proc. lenticularis des Amboss. Z. Lar. Rhinol. *59*:207 (1980).

33 Bicknell, M.R.: Bilateral traumatic interruption of the ossicular chain. J. Laryng. *80*:748–752 (1966).

34 Bicknell, P.G.: Sensorineural deafness following myringoplasty operations. J. Laryng. *85*:957–961 (1971).

35 Blohmke, A.: Die Bedeutung der Röntgenzielaufnahmen des Schläfenbeines nach Schüller, Stenvers und E.G. Mayer bei Schädelbasisbrüchen. Z. Hals-Nasen-Ohrenheilk. *29*:276–283 (1931).

36 Böhm, W.: Über Verletzung des Trommelfells durch indirekte Gewalt. Mschr. Ohrenheilk. *38*:106–111 (1904).

37 Boenninghaus, H.G.: Die Indikation zur Tympanoplastik nach Schläfenbeinlängsbruch. Arch. Ohr.-Nas.-KehlkHeilk. *173*:395–401 (1958).

38 Boenninghaus, H.G.: Die Behandlung der Schädelbasisbrüche (Thieme, Stuttgart 1960).

39 Boenninghaus, H.G.: Primäre und sekundäre Facialisparesen bei Schläfenbeinfrakturen. Z. Lar. Rhinol. *45*:325–331 (1966).

40 Boenninghaus, H.G.: Ohrverletzungen; in Berendes, Link, Zöllner, Hals-Nasen-Ohren-Heilkunde in Klinik und Praxis, Bd. V, 20.1–20.48 (Thieme, Stuttgart 1979).

41 Boenninghaus, H.G.; Gülzow, J.: Operationsindikation bei Fensterruptur und Hörsturz. Z. Lar. Rhinol. *60*:49–52 (1981).

42 Bollaert, A.; Hotton, F.; Kleiner, S.: Etude tomographique des fractures du rocher et

plus particulièrement de l'aqueduc de Fallope. J. belge Radiol. *54:*209–222 (1971).

43   Bouchayer, M.; Méréaud, P.: Fracture des branches de l'étrier par baro-traumatisme. J. fr. Oto-Rhino-Laryng. *19:*655–656 (1970).

44   Breuninger, H.; Giebel, W.: Untersuchungen über die Durchgängigkeit der Membran des runden Fensters für Tetracyclin. Arch. Oto-Rhino-Laryng. *210:*362 (1975).

45   See Munoz Borge, F.; Marco, J.: [321].

46   Brock: Spätmeningitis nach Labyrinthfraktur. Z. Hals-Nasen-Ohrenheilk. *34:*360–377 (1933).

47   Brookler, K.H.: Otitic barotrauma. Laryngoscope, St Louis *83:*966–968 (1973).

48   Brun, J.-P.; Stupp, H.; Lagler, F.; Sous, H.: Antibioticaspiegel bei lokaler Applikation verschiedener Antibiotica am Innenohr des Meerschweinchens. Arch. klin. exp. Ohr.-Nas.-KehlkHeilk. *196:*177–180 (1970).

49   Brunner, H.: The attachment of the stapes to the oval window. Archs Otolar. *59:*18–29 (1954).

50   Burton, R.D.; Lawrence, M.: Osteoblastic activity in ossicular fractures. Laryngoscope, St Louis *69:*345–357 (1959).

51   Campbell, J.: An unusual case of middle ear injury. Mich. Med. *67:* 1465–1466 (1968).

52   Carlborg, B.: On physiological and experimental variation of the perilymphatic pressure in the cat. Acta oto-lar. *91:*19–28 (1981).

53   Caruso, V.G.; Winkelmann, P.E.; Correia, M.J.; Miltenberger, G.E.; Love, J.T.: Otologic and otoneurologic injuries in divers: clinical studies on nine commercial and two sport divers. Laryngoscope, St Louis *87:*508–521 (1977).

54   Castrillo Riol, R.; Lopez Martinez, R.; Ferrandis Cardona, E.; Herrero Lacasta, E.: Sordera brusca por rotura de ventana (oval o redonda). Rev. esp. Oto-neuro-oftal. *33:*145–151 (1975).

55   Cawthorne, T.; Haynes, D.R.: Facial palsy. Br. med. J. *ii:*1197–1200 (1956).

56   Chalat, N.J.: Middle ear effects of head trauma. Laryngoscope, St Louis *81:*1286–1303 (1971).

57   Chang, H.T.; Margaria, R.; Gelfan, S.: Pressure changes and barotrauma resulting from decompression and recompression in the middle ear of monkeys. Archs Otolar. *51:*378–399 (1950).

58   Charachon, R.; Junien-Lavillauroy, C.; Dezani, M.: Fracture disjonction de l'étrier avec ankylose stapédovestibulaire, séquelle d'un traumatisme crânien grave. J. fr. Oto-Rhino-Laryng. *17:*673–677 (1968).

59   Chüden, H.G.: Ruptur der runden Fenstermembran. HNO *27:*227–231 (1979).

60   Chvojka, J.; Mrovec, J.; Siroky, J.: Traumatické subluxace a luxace trmínku. Čs. Otolaryng. *19:*233–238 (1970).

61   Chvojka, J.; Mrovec, J.: Luxation et subluxation traumatique de l'étrier. A propos de deux observations. Ann. Otolaryngol. Chir. Cervicofac. *88:*99–102 (1971).

62   Conde Jahn, F.: Barotraumatismos auriculares y sinusales. Acta oto-rhino-laring. ibero-amer. *21:*309–315 (1970).

63   Corradi, C.: Die Perforation des Trommelfells durch indirekte Ursachen, besonders vom gerichtärztlichen Standpunkt aus. Arch. Ohrenheilk. *39:*287–293 (1895).

64   Corradi, C.: Über traumatische Perforation des Trommelfells. Arch. Ohrenheilk. *43:*213 (1897).

65   Cremin, M.D.: Injuries of the ossicular chain. Z. Laryng. *83:*845–862 (1969).

66   Cummings, R.J.: Trauma. Injuries to the stapes. J. Kans. med. Soc. *77:*473–480 (1976).

67   Debrun, G.; Lacour, P.; Vinuela, F.; Fox, A.; Drake, C.G.; Caron, J.P.: Treatment of 54 traumatic carotid-cavernous fistulas. J. Neurosurg. *55:*678–692 (1981).

68a Densert, O.; Carlborg, B.; Stagg, J.: Transmission of low frequency pressure steps to the perilymphatic fluid. Acta oto-lar, *91:* 55–64 (1981).

68b Densert, O.; Ivarsson, A.; Pederson, K.: The influence of perilymphatic pressure on the displacement of the tympanic membrane. Acta oto-lar. *84:* 220–226 (1977).

69   Derlacki, E.L.: Repair of central perforations of tympanic membrane. Archs Otolar. *58:*405–420 (1953).

70   De Vos, J.; Melon, J.: Les accidents de la plongée sous-marine. Revue méd. Liège *29:*358–363 (1974).

71   Diamant, M.: Otitis and pneumatisation of the mastoid bone. Acta oto-lar. *41:*suppl., pp. 1–149 (1940).

72   Diamant, M.: Mastoid pneumatisation and its function. Archs Otolar. *76:*390–397 (1962).

73   Diamond, C.; Frew, J.: The facial nerve (Oxford University Press, London 1979).

74   Dieroff, H.-G.: Über Behandlung und Hörstörungen bei Trommelfellrupturen. HNO *10:*38–40 (1962).

75   Dietzel, K.: Erfahrungen bei der Versorgung isolierter Trommelfellverletzungen. HNO *8:*267–277 (1959/60).

76   Dietzel, K.: Über die Dehiszenzen des Facialiskanals. Z. Lar. Rhinol. *40:*366–379 (1961).

77   Dietzel, K.: Kapselplastik des Incus-Stapes-Gelenkes. Beitrag zur Sicherung der Operationsergebnisse in der Stapes-Chirurgie. Acta oto-lar. *56:*555–562 (1963).

78   Dietzel, K.: Die Mikrotraumen der ovalen Fensternische. Mschr. Ohrenheilk. *105:*174–175 (1971).

79   Dietzel, K.: Die Prädilektionsstellen von Facialisläsionen bei otobasalen Traumen. (Morpholog. u. klin. Studie). HNO-Praxis *2:*254–263 (1977).

80   Does, J.E.S.; Bottema, T.: Posttraumatic conductive hearing loss. Archs Otolar. *82:*331–339 (1965).

81   Dubreuil, C.: Lésions traumatiques de la chaîne ossiculaire. J. fr. Oto-Rhino-Laryng. *27:*489–495 (1978).

82   Dürrer, J.: Poúrazová prevodní nedoslýchavost. (Post-accidental conduction hardness of hearing.) Čs. Otolaryng. *22:*84–88 (1973).

83   Dürrer, J.: Mechanism of the laterobasal fractures. Acta oto-lar. *66:*25–32 (1968).

84   Dürrer, J.; Busek, J.: Deformations of the temporal bone in head trauma. Practica oto-rhino-lar. *31:*283–287 (1969).

85   Dürrer, J.; Busek, J.; Zemek, J.: Mechanical changes of the ossicular chain due to head injury. Practica oto-rhino-lar. *32:*293–296 (1970).

86   Dürrer, J.; Busek, J.; Zemek, J.: Biomechanické zmeny sluchových kustek pri úrazech lebky. (Biomechanical changes of the auditory ossicles after the head injury.) Čs. Otolaryng. *19:*193–194 (1970).

87   Dürrer, J.; Zemek, J.: Busek, J.: Blunt and sharp injuries to the temporal bone. ORL *36:*165–169 (1974).

88   Duken, J.: Über zwei Fälle von intrakranieller Pneumatocele nach Schussverletzung. Münch. med. Wschr. *17:*598–599 (1915).

89   Eckel, W.: Die gutachtliche Beurteilung von Ohrcholesteatomen nach Traumen. HNO *7:*235–242 (1958/59).

90 Eckel, W.: Das traumatische Cholesteatom des Gehörganges. Z. Laryng. Rhinol. *45:*265–274 (1966).

91 Eichel, B.S.; Landes, B.S.: Sensorineural hearing loss caused by skin diving. Archs Otolar. *92:*128–131 (1970).

92 Elbrond, O.: Defects of the auditory ossicles in ears with intact tympanic membrane. Clinical studies. Acta oto-lar. *264:* suppl., pp. 1–51 (1970).

93 Elbrond, O.; Aastrup, J.E.: Isolated fractures of the stapedial arch. Acta oto-lar. *75:*357–358 (1973).

94 Elner, A.; Ingelstedt, S.; Ivarsson, A.: The elastic properties of the tympanic membrane system. Acta oto-lar. *72:*397–403 (1971).

95 Elner, A.; Ingelstedt, S.; Ivarsosn, A.: A method for studies of the middle ear mechanics. Acta oto-lar. *72:*191–200 (1971).

96 Emmett, J.R.; Staab, E.V.; Fischer, N.D.: Perilymph fistulas secondary to gunshot wound. Archs. Otolar. *103:*98–102 (1977).

97 Escher, F.: Traumatische Cholesteatome. Practica oto-rhino-lar. *16:*32–40 (1954).

98 Escher, F.: Funktionelle Ohrchirurgie traumatischer Mittelohrläsionen. ORL *25:*52–53 (1963).

99 Escher, F.: Funktionelle Ohrchirurgie traumatischer Mittelohrläsionen. Adv. Oto-Rhino-Laryng., vol. 11, pp. 1–50 (Karger, Basel 1964).

100 Escher, F.: Reparative Chirurgie von Pyramidenfrakturen. Practica oto-rhino-lar. *31:*113–114 (1969).

101 Escher, F.: Reparative Chirurgie traumatischer Mittelohrläsionen. HNO *17:*65–70 (1969).

102 Escher, F.: Reparative Chirurgie traumatischer Mittelohrläsionen. Mschr. Ohrenheilk. *103:*142–144 (1969).

103 Escher, F.: Funktionelle Chirurgie des Mittelohrtraumas. HNO *18:* 359–360 (1970).

104 Escher, F.: Das Schädelbasistrauma in oto-rhinologischer Sicht. Ein Überblick über drei Jahrzehnte. HNO *21:*129–144 (1973).

105 Escher, F.: Das Trauma des Ohres. Ther. Umsch. *35:*493–501 (1978).

106 Eysell: Ist ein System gut entwickelter Warzenzellen ein Schutz gegen Ruptur des Trommelfells bei plötzlichen Luftdruckschwankungen? Arch. Ohrenheilk. *24:*75–76 (1887).

107 Fagerberg, S.; Lodin, H.: Pneumencephalus. Acta oto-lar. *58:*312–320 (1964).

108 Farmer, J.C.: Diving injuries to the inner ear. Ann. Otol., St Louis *86:* suppl. 36, pp. 1–20 (1977).

109 Fee, G.A.: Traumatic perilymphatic fistulas. Archs Otolar. *88:*477–480 (1968).

110 Femenić, B.; Subotić, R.: Zu den Tympanoplastik-Indikationen im Senium; in Kaiser-Meinhardt, Wendler, Geriatrische Aspekte in der HNO-Heilkunde, pp. 247–248 (Thieme, Leipzig 1976).

111 Fernandes, C.M.: Labyrinthine membrane rupture: a cause of post-traumatic vertigo. S. Afr. J. Surg. *15:*71–74 (1977).

112 Fisch, U.: Die totale Freilegung des Nervus facialis bei laterobasalen Schädelfrakturen. Arch. klin. exp. Ohr.-Nas.-KehlkHeilk. *196:*187–193 (1970).

113 Fisch, U.: Facial paralysis in fractures of the petrous bone. Laryngoscope, St Louis *84:*2141–2154 (1974).

114 Fisch, U.: Richtlinien zur Versorgung traumatischer Verletzungen des Nervus facialis. ORL *38:* suppl. I, pp. 42–49 (1976).

115 Fisch, U.: Facialislähmungen im labyrinthären, meatalen und intrakraniellen Bereich; in Berendes, Link, Zöllner, Hals-Nasen-Ohren-Heilkunde in Praxis und Klinik, Bd V, 21.43–21.66 (Thieme, Stuttgart 1979).

116 Fisch, U.: Management of intratemporal facial nerve injuries. J. Laryng. *94:*129–134 (1980).

117 Fleischer, K.: Das alternde Ohr: morphologische Aspekte. HNO *20:*103–107 (1972).

118 Fleischer, K.: Innenohrveränderungen nach einem stumpfen Schädeltrauma. HNO *20:*291–295 (1972).

119 Flisberg, K.: The effects of vacuum on the tympanic cavity. Otolaryngol Clin. North Am. *3:*3–13 (1970).

120 Flisberg, K.; Floberg, L.E.: Traumatic luxation of the incus in children. Acta oto-lar. *51:*469–475 (1960).

121 Flisberg, K.; Ingelstedt, S.; Örtegren, U.: Controlled 'ear aspiration' of air. Acta oto-lar. *182:* suppl., pp. 35–38 (1963).

122 Flisberg, K.; Ingelstedt, S.; Örtegren, U.: Clinical volume determination of the air-filled ear space. Acta oto-lar. *182:* suppl., pp. 39–42 (1963).

123 Flisberg, K.; Ingelstedt, S.; Örtegren, U.: On middle ear pressure. Acta oto-lar. *182:* suppl., pp. 43–56 (1963).

124 Flisberg, K.; Ingelstedt, S.; Örtegren, U.: The relationship of middle ear disease to mastoid hypocellularity. Acta oto-lar. *182:* suppl., pp. 69–72 (1963).

125 Flisberg, K.; Zsigmond, M.: The size of the mastoid air cell system. Acta oto-lar. *60:*23–29 (1965).

126 Franke, K.: Fine structure of the tissue lining the cochlear perilymphatic space against the bony labyrinthine capsule. Archs Otolar. *222:*161–167 (1979).

127 Fraser: Diskussionsbemerkung zu Nager, F.R., über Spätmeningitis nach Labyrinthfraktur. Acta oto-lar. *14:*127–134 (1930).

128 Fraser, J.G.; Harborow, P.C.: Labyrinthine window rupture. J. Laryng. *89:* 1–7 (1975).

129 Freeman, P.; Edmonds, C.: Inner ear barotrauma. Archs Otolar. *95:*556–563 (1972); cit. Freeman, P.: Inner ear barotrauma. Archs. Otolar. *97:*429 (1973).

130 Freeman, P.: Inner ear barotrauma. Archs Otolar *97:*429 (1973).

131 Freeman, P.: Rupture of the round window membrane. Acta oto-rhino-lar. belg. *29:*783–794 (1975).

132 Freeman, P.: Rupture of the round window membrane. Otolaryngol. Clin. North Am. *11:*81–93 (1978).

133 Frenkiel, S.; Alberti, P.W.: Traumatic thermal injuries of the middle ear. J. Otolaryngol. *6:*17–22 (1977).

134 Frey, K.W.: Die Tomographie bei Luxationen und Frakturen der Gehörknöchelchen. Z. Lar. Rhinol. *46:*765–775 (1967).

135 Frey, K.W.; Theopold, H.-M.: Röntgenschichtaufnahmen bei Schläfenbeinfrakturen und Verletzungen der Gehörknöchelchen. Z. Lar. Rhinol. *60:*451–470 (1981).

136 Friedman, S.I.; Sassaki, C.T.: Hearing loss during resuscitation. Archs Otolar. *101:*385–386 (1975).

137 Gaillard, J.; Haguenauer, J.P.; Romanet, P.; Dubreuil, C.: Traumatisme crânien: luxation à distance de l'enclume et lésions multiples de l'oreille moyenne. J. fr. Oto-Rhino-Laryng. *27:*357–359 (1978).

138 Glaninger, J.: Untersuchungen zur Festigkeit der Gehörknöchelchen und ihrer Gelenke. Mschr. Ohrenheilk. *95:*353–375 (1961).

139 Glaninger, J.: Zur operativen Behandlung von traumatischen Läsionen der Ossicula auditus. Mschr. Ohrenheilk. *103:*340–350 (1969).

140 Goodhill, V.: Deliberate 'spontaneous' tympanoplasty: roles of annular induction and basement membranes. Ann. Otol., St Louis *75:*866–880 (1966).

141 Goodhill, V.: Sudden deafness and round window rupture. Laryngoscope, St Louis *81:*1462–1474 (1971).

142 Goodhill, V.: Labyrinthine membrane ruptures in sudden sensorineural hearing loss. Proc. R. Soc. Med. *69:*565–572 (1976).

143 Goodhill, V.:Traumatic fistulae. J. Laryng. *94:*123–128 (1980).

144 Goodhill, V.: Leaking labyrinth lesions, deafness, tinnitus and dizziness. Ann. Otol., St Louis *90:*99–105 (1981).

145 Goodhill, V.; Brockman, S.J.; Harris, I.; Hantz. O.: Sudden deafness and labyrinthine window ruptures. Audiovestibular observations. Ann. Otol., St Louis *82:* 2–12 (1973).

146 Goodman, P.M.; Morioka, W.T.: Round window membrane rupture. Laryngoscope, St Louis *88:*383–388 (1978).

147 Grahe, K.: Abnorme Cholesteatombildung am Felsenbein. Z. Lar. Rhinol. *20:*133–135 (1931).

148 Gray, R.F.; Barton, R.P.E.: Round window rupture. J. Laryng. *95:*165–177 (1981).

149 Grete, W.: Geheilter Temporallappenabszess nach Felsenbeinfraktur. Arch. Ohrenheilk. *131:*245–264 (1932).

150 Griffin, W.L., jr.: A retrospective study of traumatic tympanic membrane perforations in a clinical practice. Laryngoscope, St Louis *89:*261–282 (1979).

151 Grimaud, R.; Perrin, C.; Richardin, C.: Les brûlures tympaniques. Incertitudes pronostiques. Difficultés thérapeutiques. Ann. Otolaryngol. Chir. Cervicofac. *88:*143–149 (1971).

152 Gros, J.C.: The ear in skull trauma. Sth. med. J., Nashville *60:*705–711 (1967).

153 Grove, W.E.: Skull fractures involving the ear; clinical study of 211 cases. Part I. Laryngoscope, St Louis *49:*678–707 (1939).

154 Grove, W.E.: Skull fractures involving the ear; clinical study of 211 cases. Part II. Laryngoscope, St Louis *49:*833–867 (1939).

155 Gruber, J.: Lehrbuch der Ohrenheilkunde (Gerold's Sohn, Wien 1870).

156 Grundfast, K.M.; Bluestone, C.D.: Sudden or fluctuating hearing loss and vertigo in children due to perilymph fistula. Ann. Otol., St Louis *87:*761–771 (1978).

157 Guennel, F.: Operationsbefunde und -Ergebnisse nach traumatischer Zerstörung der Gehörknöchelchenkette und Schädigung des N. facialis. Z. ärztl. Fortbild. *60:*250–251 (1966).

158 Guerrier, Y.: Lésions traumatiques des osselets. Le mécanisme des lésions ossiculaires dans les traumatismes fermés du crâne. Acta oto-rhino-lar. belg. *25:*606–614 (1971).

159 Guerrier, Y.: Le point de vue de l'anatomiste sur les liquorrhées cérébrospinales. 2e Coll. ORL de Foch, pp. 9–16, 1978.

160 Guerrier, Y.; Grado, F. de; Guerrier, B.: Les traumatismes de l'oreille moyenne. Urgences chirurgicales. Cah. Oto-rhino-laryng. *11:*601–606 (1976).

161 Guerrier, Y.; Dejean, Y.; Galy, G.: Les surdités de transmission dans les traumatismes fermés du crâne. Cah. Oto-rhino-laryng. *1:*11–66 (1965/66).

162 Guerrier, Y.; Dejan, Y.; Serrou, B.: Le traitement chirurgical des traumatismes de l'oreille moyenne (à propos de 109 observations). Revue Laryng., Bordeaux *88:*903–915 (1967).

163 Guerrier, Y.; Dejan, Y.; Serrou, B.: Lésions de l'oreille moyenne, paralysies faciales exceptées, après traumatismes crâniens fermés. J. fr. Oto-Rhino-Lar. *17:*123–128 (1968).

164 Guerrier, Y.; Guerrier, B.: Les luxations traumatiques de l'enclume. Arch. Ital. oto-rino-laring. *7:*177–187 (1979).

165 Güttich, H.: Trommelfellverbrennung ohne Gehörgangsverbrennung bei Schweissern und Eisenbrennern. HNO *7:*273–274 (1959).

166 Gundersen, T.; Molvaer, O.I.: Hearing loss resulting from perilymph fistula. A presentation of two cases. Acta oto-lar. *85:*324–327 (1978).

167 Gussen, R.: Round window niche melanocytes and webby tissue. Archs Otolar. *104:*662–668 (1978).

168 Gussen, R.: Sudden hearing loss associated with cochlear membrane rupture. Archs. Otolar. *107:*598–600 (1981).

169 Haguenauer, J.P.; Gaillard, J.; Dumolard, P.; Grégoire, D.: Méningocèle atticale post-traumatique. J. fr. Oto-Rhino-Lar. *24:*635–636 (1975).

170 Hahlbrock, K.H.: Versorgung frischer Trommelfellverletzungen. Arch. Ohr.-Nas.-KehlkHeilk. *171:*120–127 (1958).

171 Hahlbrock, K.H.: Die mikrochirurgische Versorgung von Trommelfellverletzungen. Z. Lar. Rhinol. *45:*286–292 (1966).

172 Hamberger, C.A.; Wersäll, J.: Vascular supply of the tympanic membrane and ossicular chain. Acta oto-lar. *188:* suppl., pp. 308–318 (1964).

173 Hammond, V.T.: Ossicular lesions. J. Laryng. *94:*117–122 (1980)

174 Hanneuse, Y.; Mestrez. F.: A propos de deux cas d'otoliquorrhée. Acta oto-rhino-lar. belg. *30:*325–333 (1976).

175 Harker, L.A.; Norante, J.D.; Ryu, J.H.: Round window bulging and blowout on increased cerebro-spinal fluid pressure. Trans. Am. Acad. Ophthal. Oto-lar. *77:*447 (1973).

176 Hartmann, A.: Die Krankheiten des Ohres (Fischer, Berlin 1892).

177 Haymann, L.: Über Schussverletzungen des Ohres. Teil 1. Zentbl. Ohrenheilk. *13:*127–149 (1915).

178 Haymann, L.: Über Schussverletzungen des Ohres. Teil 2. Zentbl. Ohrenheilk. *13:*159–168 (1915).

179 Haymann, L.: Über Schussverletzungen des Ohres. Teil 3. Zentbl. Ohrenheilk. *16:*1–8 (1919).

180 Haymann, L.: Über Schussverletzungen des Ohres. Teil 4. Zentbl. Ohrenheilk. *16:*33–42 (1919).

181 Haymann, L.: Über Schussverletzungen des Ohres. Teil 5. Zentbl. Ohrenheilk. *16:*65–83 (1919).

182 Head, P.W.: Decompression injuries in the temporal bone. J. Laryng. *94:*111–116 (1980).

183 Healy, G.B.; Friedman, J.M.; Strong, M.S.: Vestibular and auditory findings of perilymph fistula. A review of 40 cases. Trans. Am. Acad. Ophthal. Oto-lar. *88:*44–49 (1976).

184 Healy, G.B.; Strong, M.S.; Sampogna, D.: Ataxia, vertigo, and hearing loss. A result of rupture of inner ear window. Archs Otolar. *100:*130–135 (1974).

185 Heermann, J.; Dammad, H.; Spernau, H.: Perilymphschwall aus Perforation des runden Fensters nach leichtem Schädeltrauma bei vermutlich weitem Aquaeductus cochleae. Z. Lar. Rhinol. *55:*549–550 (1976).

186 Heermann, O.: Über einige Fälle von Gehörgangs- Mittelohr- und Labyrinthverbren-
     nungen beim Schweissen und Giessen. Z. Hals-Nasen-Ohrenheilk. *39:*546–556 (1936).
187 Helms, J.: Experimentelle und klinische Untersuchungen zur Funktion des normalen,
     erkrankten und operierten Trommelfells; Habil.-schrift, Tübingen (1975).
188 Helms, J.: The transmeatal approach to the geniculate ganglion. Acta oto-rhino-lar.
     belg. *30:*84–89 (1976).
189 Helms, J.: Facialistraumen am Ganglion geniculi. Z. Lar. Rhinol. *58:*144–148 (1979).
190 Hermann, N.: Experimentelle und casuistische Studien über Frakturen der Schädel-
     basis; Inaug.-Diss., Dorpat (1881).
191 Herrmann, R.: Die Prognose der Spontanheilung bei Trommelfellverletzungen. Z. Lar.
     Rhinol. *45:*283–286 (1966).
192 Hildmann, H.: Die Diagnostik der laterobasalen Fraktur. Dt. med. Wschr.
     *97:*1034–1035 (1972).
193 Hildmann, H.; Steinbach, E.: Experimental studies on closing of artificial eardrum per-
     forations in rabbits. J. Laryng. *85:*1173–1176 (1971).
194 Hociota, D.: Miringoplastia prin stimularea autorefacerii timpanului. Revue Chir. (Oto-
     rinolaryngol.) *19:*341–345 (1974).
195 Hociota, D.; Ataman, T.; Apostol, N.; Solomon, S.: Unele consideratii asupra trauma-
     tismelor accidentale ossiculare. Revue Chir. (Otorinolaryngol.) *20:*29–36 (1975).
196 Höfling, O.: Lehrbuch der Physik. Oberstufe, Ausg. A., S. 257–264 (Dümmler, Han-
     nover 1959).
197 Höft, J.: Elektronenmikroskopische Untersuchungen über die Durchlässigkeit der
     Membran des runden Fensters beim Meerschweinchen. Arch. klin. exp. Ohr.-Nas.-
     KehlkHeilk. *191:*539–540 (1968).
198 Hörbst, L.: Über das primäre Cholesteatom des äusseren Gehörganges. Mschr. Ohren-
     heilk. *98:*143–154 (1964).
199 Holler, F.C.; Greenberg, L.M.: Incudostapedial joint disarticulation. Archs Otolar.
     *95:*182–184 (1972).
200 Holmquist, J.: Size of mastoid air cell system in relation to healing after myringoplasty
     and to Eustachian tube function. Acta oto-lar. *69:*89–93 (1970).
201 Hooper, R.E.; Ruben, R.J.; Mahmood, K.: Gunshot injuries of the temporal bone.
     Archs Otolar. *96:*433–440 (1972).
202 Hough, J.V.D.: Restoration of hearing loss after head trauma. Ann. Otol., St Louis
     *78:*210–226 (1969).
203 Hough, J.V.D.: Surgical aspects of temporal bone fractures. Proc. R. Soc. Med.
     *63:*245–252 (1970).
204 Hough, J.V.D.; Stuart, W.D.: Middle ear injuries in skull trauma. Laryngoscope, St
     Louis *78:*899–937 (1968).
205 House, W.F.; Crabtree, J.A.: Surgical exposure of petrous portion of seventh nerve.
     Archs Otolar. *81:*506–507 (1965).
206 Howard, M.L.: Complete round-window fistula. Ear Nose Throat J. *55:*382–383 (1976).
207 Hsu, W.C.: Garlic slice in repairing eardrum perforation. Chin. med. J. *3:*204–205
     (1977).
208 Ilberg, C. v.: Die Innenohrschwerhörigkeit nach stumpfem Schädeltrauma. Z. Lar. Rhi-
     nol. *56:*323–328 (1977).
209 Imhofer, R.: Gerichtliche Ohrenheilkunde (Kabitzsch, Leipzig 1920).
210 Ingelstedt, S.; Örtegren, U.: Qualitative testing of the Eustachian tube function. Acta
     oto-lar. *182:* suppl., pp. 7–23 (1963).

211 Ingelstedt, S.; Örtegren, U.: The ear snorkel-pressure chamber technique. Acta oto-lar. *182:* suppl., pp. 24–34 (1963).

212 Ivarsson, A.; Pedersen, K.: Volume-pressure properties of round and oval window. Acta oto-lar. *84:*38–43 (1977).

213 Jackson, P.D.: Traumatic ossicular discontinuity with stapes fixation. J. Laryng. *90:*707–709 (1976).

214 Jensen, J.; Thomsen, J.: Dislocation of the incus. The reliability of tomography. Arch. klin. exp. Ohr.-Nas.-KehlkHeilk. *204:*143–149 (1973).

215 Jensma, H.: Acute labyrinth-window rupture. Clin. Otolaryngol. *4:*474 (1979).

216 Johnson, J.K.; Sasaki, C.T.; Yanagisawa, E.: Fluctuating posttraumatic hearing loss. Ear Nose Throat J. *55:*328–330 (1976).

217 Jongkees, L.B.W.: Facial paralysis complicating skull trauma. Archs Otolar. *81:*518–522 (1965).

218 Jordan, L.: Traumatic rupture of the tympanic membrane. Laryngoscope, St Louis *62:*615–622 (1952).

219 Juers, A.L.: Office closure of tympanic perforations: a new approach. Laryngoscope, St Louis *68:*1207–1215 (1958).

220 Juers, A.L.: Perforation closure by marginal eversion. Archs Otolar. *77:*76–80 (1963).

221 Juers, A.L.: Traumatic tympanic perforation. Trans. Am. Acad. Ophthal. Oto-lar. *78:*261–263 (1974).

222 Jungmayr, H.: Fraktur des Hammergriffs mit Pseudarthrose nach stumpfem Schädeltrauma. HNO *4:*277 (1954).

223 Jungmayr, H.: Cholesteatomentstehung nach Felsenbeinfraktur. Z. Lar. Rhinol. *36:*365–368 (1957).

224 Junien-Lavillauroy, C.; Serero, C.; Charachon, R.: Fracture pathologique de l'enclume. J. fr. Oto-Rhino-Laryng. *22:*59–61 (1973).

225 Karrenstein: Über Schädigungen des Gehörorgans im Minenkrieg. Beitr. Anat. etc., Ohr *8:*271–283 (1916).

226 Kawabata, J.; Paparella, M.M.: Fine structure of the round window membrane. Ann. Otol., St Louis *80:*13–26 (1971).

227 Kecht, B.: Defektplastik bei Hirn-Dura-Prolaps in die Mittelohrräume. Arch. Ohr.-Nas.-KehlkHeilk. *174:*470–485 (1960).

228 Kecht, B.: Mittelohrverödung bei kompletter Ausschaltung, speziell nach Schläfenbeinfrakturen. Mschr. Ohrenheilk. *95:*214–221 (1961).

229 Kelemen, G.: Traumatische Cholesteatomgenese. Acta oto-lar. *20:*211–230 (1934).

230 Kelemen, G.: Fractures of the temporal bone. Archs Otolar. *40:*333–373 (1944).

231 Keller, P.A., jr.: A study of the relationship of air pressure to myringorupture. Laryngoscope, St Louis *68:*2015–2029 (1958).

232 Kerr, A.G.: Blast injuries to the ear. Practitioner *221:*677–682 (1978).

233 Kerr, A.G.: Trauma and the temporal bone. J. Laryng. *94:*107–110 (1980).

234 Kerth, J.D.; Allen, G.W.: Comparison of the perilymphatic and cerebro-spinal fluid pressures. Archs Otolar. *77:*581–585 (1963).

235 Kettel, K.: Chirurgische Wiederherstellung gegenüber abwartender Haltung in Fällen von traumatischer Facialislähmung. Arch. Ohr.-Nas.-KehlkHeilk. *180:* 444–456 (1962).

236 Kettel, K.: Surgery of the facial nerve. Archs Otolar. *81:*523–526 (1965).

237 Khan, N.A.: Zur operativen Behandlung der traumatischen Trommelfellperforation. HNO *21:*363–364 (1973).

238 Khan, N.A.: New method for the treatment of traumatic eardrum perforations. Acta oto-rhino-lar. belg. *28:*623–626 (1974).

239 Kiesselbach, W.: Die Fremdkörper im Ohre; in Schwartze, Handbuch der Ohrenheilkunde, Bd II, S. 555–569 (Vogel, Leipzig 1893).

240 King, P.F.: Aural problems in the armed services : otitic barotrauma and related conditions. Proc. R. Soc. Med. *68:*817–818 (1975).

241 King, P.F.: Otic batrotrauma. Audiology *15:*279–286 (1976).

242 Kirikae, I.; Matsuzaki, C.; Fujita, S.: 4 cases of ossicular chain disorders due to head injury. Otolaryngology, Tokyo *39:*363–373 (1967).

243 Kittel, G.: Traumatische, intrakranielle Luftansammlungen. Z. Lar. Rhinol. *39:* 234–242 (1960).

244 Kleinfeldt, D.: Defekte des runden Fensters beim akuten Hörverlust und ihre operative Therapie durch Membranplastik. HNO-Praxis *3:*38–46 (1978).

245 Kleinfeldt, D.; Dahl, D.: Zur Druckbelastung der runden Fenstermembran der Cochleae im Tierversuch. HNO-Praxis *4:*193–195 (1979).

246 Kleinschmidt, E.G.; Vick, U.: Proteinstudie zur Frage der Perilymphsubstitution durch Liquor cerebro-spinalis via aquaeductus cochleae. Acta oto-lar. *82:* 99–105 (1976).

247 Klestadt, A.: Spätmeningitis nach Labyrinthfraktur. Verh. dt. otol. Ges. *22:*229–245 (1913).

248 Kley, W.: Frakturen und Luxationen der Gehörknöchelchenkette bei Schläfenbeinfrakturen. Z. Lar. Rhinol. *45:*292–313 (1966).

249 Kley, W.: Die Unfallchirurgie der Schädelbasis und der pneumatischen Räume. Arch. Ohr.-Nas.-KehlkHeilk. *191:*1–216 (1968).

250 Klingenberg, A.: Die isolierte Schneckenfraktur bei Schädelbasisbrüchen. Z. Hals-Nasen-Ohrenheilk. *22:*452–463 (1929).

251 Knight, N.J.: Severe sensorineural deafness in children due to perforation of the round-window membrane. Lancet *ii:* 1002–1005 (1977).

252 Knight, N.J.; Phillips, M.J.: Round window membrane and aquired sensori-neural hearing loss in children. Clin. Otolaryngol. *5:*117–128 (1980).

253 Kobrak, H.G.: Untersuchungen über den Zusammenhang zwischen Hirndruck und Labyrinthdruck. Z. Hals-Nasen-Ohrenheilk. *34:*456–463 (1933).

254 Kobrak, H.G.: Round window membrane of the cochlea (experiments demonstrating its physical responses). Archs Otolar. *49:*36–47 (1949).

255 Korkis, F.B.: Rupture of the tympanic membrane of blast origin. J. Laryng. *61:*367–390 (1946).

256 Krekorian, E.A.: The repair of combat-injured facial nerves. Laryngoscope, St Louis *81:*1926–1945 (1971).

257 Kreyszig, E.: Statistische Methoden und ihre Anwendung (Vandenhoeck & Ruprecht, Göttingen 1967).

258 Kuruma, K.; Sakurai, S.; Sasaki, J.; Kawashiro, N.: Hot-water burn of the ear drum. Otolaryngology, Tokyo *41:*951–955 (1969).

259 Kuschke, E.: Conductive deafness following head injury: repair of a dislocated incudostapedial joint by wiring. S. Afr. med. J. *43:*42–44 (1969).

260 Kuschke, E.: Incudostapedial joint disarticulation. Archs Otolar. *96:*290 (1972).

261 Lamkin, R.; Axelsson, A.; McPherson, D.; Miller, J.: Experimental aural barotrauma. Electrophysiological and morphological findings. Acta oto-lar. *335:* suppl., pp. 1–24 (1975).

262 Lange, W.: Beiträge zur pathologischen Anatomie der Verletzungen des Gehörorganes. Beitr. Anat. etc., Ohr *18:*277–304 (1922).

263 Langenbeck, B.: Konservative Tympanoplastik. Z. Lar. Rhinol. *37:*118–124 (1958).

264 Leonard, J.R.; Belafsky, M.L.: Temporal bone fractures: three identical cases of lateral middle ear fractures with facial nerve injury and conductive hearing loss. Laryngoscope, St Louis *83:*587–593 (1973).

265 Lesoine, W.: Ambossfraktur nach Ohrspülung ohne Trommelfellverletzung. Z. Lar. Rhinol. *48:*352–355 (1969).

266 Linck, A.: Beitrag zur Kenntnis der Ohrverletzungen bei Schädelbasisfraktur. Z. Ohren-heilk. *57:*7–22 (1909).

267 Linck, A.: Die Zuständigkeit der Oto-Rhinologie bei der Beurteilung und Behandlung von Verletzungen im Gebiet der vorderen und seitlichen Schädelbasis. Z. Ohrenheilk. *79:*165–189 (1920).

268 Lindeman, H.: Some histological examinations of the incus and stapes with especial regard to their vascularization. Acta oto-lar. *188:* suppl., pp. 319–326 (1964).

269 Lindsay, J.R.; Zajtchuk, J.: Concussion of the inner ear. Ann. Otol., St Louis *79:*699–709 (1970).

270 Link, R.: Beitrag zur Histologie der Membran des runden Fensters. Hals-Nas.-Ohrenarzt *32:*295–302 (1942).

271 Lion, H.: Isolierte Trommelfellverbrennung. Arch. Ohr.-Nas.-KehlkHeilk. *122:*195–197 (1929).

272 Love, J.T.; Caruso, V.G.: Civilian air travel and the otolaryngologist. Laryngoscope, St Louis *88:*1732–1742 (1978).

273 Love, J.T.; Waguespack, R.W.: Perilymphatic fistulas. Laryngoscope, St Louis *91:*1118–1128 (1981).

274 Lundin, K.; Ridell, A.; Sandberg, N.; Öhmann, A.: One thousand maxillo-facial and related fractures at the ENT-clinic in Gothenburg. Acta oto-lar. *75:*359–361 (1973).

275 Lyons, G.D.; Dodson, M.L.; Casey, D.A.; Melancon, B.B.: Round window rupture secondary to acoustic trauma. Sth. med. J. Nashville *71:*71–73 (1978).

278 McCracken, D.: Traumatic rupture of ear drum. Br. med. J. 1133–1134 (1976).

279 McGibbon, J.E.G.: Aviation pressure deafness. J. Laryng. *57:*14–22 (1942).

280 McGibbon, J.E.G.: The nature of the valvular action (passive opening) of the Eusta-chian tube in relation to changes of atmospheric pressure and to aviation pressure deaf-ness. J. Laryng. *57:*344–350 (1942).

281 McIntire, G.; Benitez, J.T.: Spontaneous repair of the tympanic membrane. Histopath-ological studies in the cat. Ann. Otol., St Louis *79:*1129–1131 (1970).

282 McNicoll, W.D.: Traumatic perforation of the tympanic membrane with associated rupture of the round window membrane. J. Laryng. *92:*897–903 (1978).

283 McReynolds, G.; Guildford, F.; Chase, G.: Blast injuries to the ear. Archs Otolar. *50:*1–8 (1949).

284 Maddox, H.E.; Kosoy, J.: Traumatic labyrinthine fistula. Ann. Otol., St Louis *79:*633–640 (1970).

285 Manasse, P.: Schädelbasisfraktur und Otitis media. Beitr. Anat. etc., Ohr *21:*230–235 (1924).

286 Manasse, P.: Zur pathologischen Anatomie der traumatischen Taubheit. Vichows Arch. *189:*188–209 (1907).

287 Marquet, J.: Considérations sur le diagnostic des surdités de transmission par trauma-tisme de l'oreille. Acta oto-rhino-lar. belg. *25:*641–652 (1971).

288 Martin, H.; Gignoux, B.; Oudot, J.; Chalard, R.; Des brûlures du tympan et de la caisse. J. fr. Oto-Rhino-Laryng. *21:*885–889 (1972).

289 Martin, H.; Martin, C.: Paralysies faciales par luxations traumatiques de l'enclume. I. J. fr. Oto-Rhino-Laryng. *26:*525–526 (1977).

290 Martin, H.; Martin, C.: Paralysies faciales par luxations traumatiques de l'enclume. II. J. fr. Oto-Rhino-Laryng. *26:*529–532 (1977).

291 Martin, H.; Martin, C.; Elbaz, R.: A propos de la fermeture osseuse spontanée de certaines fenestrations platinaires. J. fr. Oto-Rhino-Lar. *30:*581–583 (1981).

292 Martins, M.: Symptomatologie und Therapie der Stapesimpression und Stapesluxation. HNO *24:*396–398 (1976).

293 Meier, D.; Büsch, F.: Cochleovestibuläre Störungen nach Tauchunfällen. ORL *38:* suppl. I, pp. 62–65 (1976).

294 Messerer, O.: Über Elasticität und Festigkeit der menschlichen Knochen (Cotta, Stuttgart 1880).

295 Messerer, O.: Experimentelle Untersuchungen über Schädelbrüche (Rieger, München 1884).

296 Messervy, M.: Unilateral ossicular disruption following blast exposure. Laryngoscope, St Louis *82:*372–375 (1972).

297 Miehlke, A.: Intracranial facial nerve repair (Dott's operation). Archs Otolar. *81:*507–508 (1965).

298 Miehlke, A.: Surgery of the facial nerve (Urban & Schwarzenberg, München 1973).

299 Miehlke, A.; Fisch, U.: Facialislähmungen; in Berendes, Link, Zöllner, Hals-Nasen-Ohren-Heilkunde in Praxis und Klinik, Bd V, 21.1–21.66 (Thieme, Stuttgart 1979).

300 Minami, Y.; Nakamura, H.: 2 cases of fracture of the inner ear. Otolaryngology, Tokyo *42:*663–667 (1970).

301 Minnigerode, B.; Küpper, R.; Karduck, A.; Bartholomé, W.: Der ohrenärztliche Frühbefund bei Schädelverletzten. Unfallheilk. *79:*439–442 (1976).

302 Miriszlai, E.; Benedeczky, J.; Csapó, S.; Bodánszky, H.: The ultrastructure of the round window membrane of the cat. ORL *40:*111–119 (1978).

303 Miriszlai, E.; Sandor, P.: Investigations on the critical perilymphatic pressure value causing round window membrane rupture in anesthetized cats. Acta oto-lar. *89:*323–329 (1980).

304 Möbius, M.: Schweissperlenverletzungen des Trommelfelles. HNO *12:*18–22 (1964).

305 Mölling: Diskussionsbemerkung. HNO *1:*137 (1948).

306 Molvaer, O.I.; Eidsvik, S.: Dykking og skade av det indre yret. Tidsskr. norske. Laegeforen. *98:*263–265 (1978).

307 Molvaer, O.I.; Natrud, E.; Eidsvik, S.: Diving injuries to the inner ear. Archs Otolar. *221:*285–288 (1978).

308 Molvaer, O.I.; Vallersnes, F.M.; Kringlebotn, M.: The size of the middle ear and the mastoid air cell system measured by an acoustic method. Acta oto-lar. *85:*24–32 (1978).

309 Montandon, P.: Fistules traumatiques de la fenêtre ovale avec épanchement de liquide céphalo-rachidien. Revue Oto-Neuro-Ophthal. *47:*419–421 (1975).

310 Morgon, A.; Charachon, R.: Aspects cliniques de l'otite barotraumatique en plongée sous-marine. J. fr. Oto-Rhino-Laryng. *24:*609–611 (1975).

311 Moritsch, E.: Zur chirurgischen Therapie erworbener Gehörgangsstenosen. Z. Laryng. Rhinol. *56:*800–804 (1977).

312 Morizono, T.: Study of experimental deafness with particular reference ot the ototoxic substances and altered cochlear circulation; Habil.-Schrift, Univ. W.-Australien (1975).

313 Mosher, W.F.: Foreign bodies of external canal, middle ear and mastoid and their complications. Archs Otolar. *36:*679–686 (1942).

314 Mostafa, H.: The recent conceptions of traumatic perforations of the tympanic membrane with a record of twenty cases. J. Egypt. med. Ass. *49:*271–274 (1966).

315 Mounier-Kuhn, P.; Morgan, A.; Bouchayer, M.: Les séquelles des traumatismes directs du tympan. Revue Laryng., Bordeaux *88:*849–853 (1967).

316 Moure, E.J.: Fracture probable des osselets de l'ouie par violence indirecte. Arch. Ohrenheilk. *21:*203–204 (1884).

317 Müller, A.H.; Edel, P.: Röntgenologische Aspekte der Felsenbeinfrakturen mit Facialisparese. ORL *38:* suppl. 1, pp. 36–41 (1976).

318 Mündnich, K.: Die Schussverletzungen des Ohres und der seitlichen Schädelbasis (Thieme, Leipzig 1944).

319 Münker, G.: Personal communication (1981).

320 Mullan, S.; Duda, E.E.; Patrona,s N.J.: Some examples of balloon technology in neurosurgery. J. Neurosurg. *52:*321–329 (1980).

321 Munoz Borge, F.; Marco, J.: Traumatismos de la cadena osicular. Acta oto-rino-laring. ibero-amer. *23:*279–282 (1972).

322 Murphy, K.W.: Head injury and fractures of the ankylosed stapes. J. Laryng. *86:*169–171 (1972).

323 Myers, P.W.: Jugular vein compression and elevation of perilymphatic fluid pressure. Archs Otolar. *98:*314–315 (1973).

324 Nager, F.R.: Über Spätmeningitis nach Labyrinthfraktur. Arch. Ohrenheilk. *122:*217–229 (1929).

325 Nager, F.R.: Über Spätmeningitis nach Labyrinthfraktur. Acta oto-lar. *14:*127–134 (1930).

326 Nakano, Y.; Ishikawa, K.: Stapedial fracture following head trauma. Otolaryngology, Tokyo *41:*113–117 (1969).

327 Nedzelski, J.M.; Barber, H.O.: Round window fistula. J. Otolaryngol. *5:*379–385 (1976).

328 Nejedlo, V.: Zur Frage des spontanen Verschlusses der zentralen Trommelfelldefekte. Z. Lar. Rhinol. *48:*855–864 (1969).

329 Nilsson, G.: Attic cholesteatoma following longitudinal fracture of the pyramid. Acta oto-lar. *36:*85–91 (1948).

330 Nishimura, S.; Yanagita, N.; Inafuku, S.; Handoh, M.; Yokoi, H.; Futatsugi, Y.; Miyake, H.: A scanning electron microscopic study of the guinea pig cochlear aqueduct. ORL *43:*79–88 (1981).

331 Okuneff, W.N.: Über die Anwendung des Acidum trichloraceticum bei chronischen eitrigen Entzündungen des Mittelohres. Mschr. Ohrenheilk. *29:*1–14 (1895).

332 Ombredanne, M.: Absence congénitale de fenêtre ronde dans certaines aplasies mineures. Annls Oto-lar. *85:*369–378 (1968).

333 Oppenheimer, P.; Kaplan, J.; Harrison, W.; Gandhi, K.: Repair of traumatic myringorupture. Archs Otolar. *73:*328–333 (1961).

334 Owens, W.D.; Gustave, F.; Sclaroff, A.: Tympanic membrane rupture with nitrous oxide anesthesia. Anesth. Analg., Cleveland *57:*283–286 (1978).

335 Pahor, A.L.: Tympanic membrane epidermoid following head injury. Ear Nose Throat J. *57:*330–332 (1978).

336 Pahor, A.L.: The ENT problems following the Birmingham bombings. J. Laryng. *95:*399–406 (1981).

337 Palva, T.; Dammert, K.: Human cochlear aqueduct. Acta oto-lar. *246:* suppl., pp. 1–58 (1969).

338 Pang, L.Q.: The otological aspects of whiplash injuries. Laryngoscope, St Louis *81:*1381–1387 (1971).

339 Passow, A.: Die Verletzungen des Gehörorganes (Bergmann, Wiesbaden 1905).

340 Passow. A.: Über Luftansammlung im Schädelinnern. Beitr. Anat. etc., Ohr *8:*257–270 (1916).

341 Patterson, M.E.; Bartlett, P.C.: Hearing impairment caused by intratympanic pressure changes during general anesthesia. Laryngoscope, St Louis *86:*399–404 (1976).

342 Pellegrini, G.; Firmas, J.L. de : Ecoulement de liquide céphalo-rachidien consécutif à l'ouverture des fenêtres labyrinthiques par blast liquidien. Revue Laryng., Bordeaux *91:*597–601 (1970).

343 Pellerin, J.; Poncet, P.: Fracture de la platine de l'étrier par traumatisme direct. Ann. Oto-laryngol. Chir. cervicofac. (Paris) *94:*520–525 (1977).

344 Perlman, H.B.: The Eustachian tube: Abnormal patency and normal physiologic state. Arch. Otolaryng. *30:*212–238 (1939).

345 Piquet, J.-J.: Les oto-liquorrhées post-traumatiques. 2è coll. ORL de Foch, pp. 39–44 (1978).

346 Plath, P.: Fraktur und Luxation des Amboss nach Schädeltraumen bei Otosklerose. HNO *16:*59 (1968).

347 Plester, D.: Ambossluxation und Reposition. Arch. Ohr.-Nas.-Kehlk Heilk. *171:* 137 (1957).

348 Plester, D.: Die operative Behandlung der Gehörknöchelchenluxationen. Z. Lar. Rhinol. *38:*221–225 (1959).

349 Plester, D.: Das alternde Ohr: chirurgische Aspekte. HNO *20:*216–217 (1972).

350 Politzer, A.: Lehrbuch der Ohrenheilkunde (Enke, Stuttgart 1887).

351 Portmann, M.: Management of ossicular chain defects. J. Laryng. *81:*1309–1323 (1967).

352 Proctor, B.; Gurdjian, E.S.; Webster, J.E.: The ear in head trauma. Laryngoscope, St Louis *66:*16–59 (1956).

353 Pullen, F.W.: Round window membrane rupture: a cause of sudden deafness. Trans. Am. Acad. Ophthal. Oto-lar. *76:*1444–1450 (1972).

354 Rask-Andersen, H.; Stahle, J.; Wilbrand, H.: Human cochlear aqueduct and its accessory canals. Ann. Otol., St Louis *86:* suppl. 42, pp. 1–16 (1977).

355 Reeve, D.R.: Repair of large experimental perforations of the tympanic membrane. J. Laryng. *91:*767–778 (1977).

356 Reijnen, C.J.; Kuijpers, W.: The healing pattern of the drum membrane. Acta oto-lar. *287:* suppl., pp. 1–74 (1971).

357 Rettinger, G.: Gehörgangsreinigung mit Wattestäbchen — Sinn oder Unsinn? Dt. Ärzteblatt. *26:*1447–1450 (1979).

358 Richardson, T.L.; Ishiyama, E.; Keels, E.W.: Submicroscopic studies of the round window membrane. Acta oto-lar. *71:*9–21 (1971).

359 Robinson, M.: The diagnosis and management of injuries of the ossicular chain. Eye Ear Nose Throat Mon. *48:*689–692 (1969).

360 Roche, J.: Fractures of the temporal bone involving the ear. Australas. Radiol. *19:*317–325 (1975).

361 Rohrt, T.: Fracture of temporal bone, early or retrospective diagnosis and surgical hearing reconstruction. Acta oto-lar. *75:*355–356 (1973).

362 Roithner, H.: Durch Gehörknöchelchenverletzung maskierte otosklerotische Schwerhörigkeit. Mschr. Ohrenheilk. *107:* 1–5 (1973).

363 Rothman, W.; Matta, I.; Cole, J.M.: Transtympanic facial nerve paralysis. Trans. Pa. Acad. Ophthal. Otolaryng. *30:* 45–48 (1977).

364 Rudert, H.; Haddad, H.: Thermisches Trauma des Hörorgans. HNO *19:* 309–311 (1971).

365 Rüedi, R.; Furrer, W.: Das akustische Trauma. Practica oto-rhino-lar. *8:* 177–372 (1946).

366 Ruggles, R.L.; Votypka, R.: Blast injuries of the ear. Laryngoscope, St Louis *83:* 974–976 (1973).

367 Rumler: Über Regeneration und Narbenbildung des Trommelfells. Arch. Ohrenheilk. *30:* 142–157 (1890).

368 Sadé, J.: Traumatic fractures of the stapes. Archs Otolar. *80:* 258–262 (1964).

369 Sakai, K.: Anatomische Befunde am menschlichen Gehörorgan nach Basisfraktur. Arch. Ohrenheilk. *85:* 188–197 (1911).

370 Samuel, E.: Radiological investigation of injuries of the temporal bone. Proc. R. Soc. Med. *63:* 252–256 (1970).

371 Schein, G.C.: Thermal effects on the tympanic membrane. Laryngoscope, St Louis *65:* 1043–1056 (1955).

372 Schlittler, E.: Labyrinthzersplitterung-isolierte Vestibularfraktur-Spätmeningitis nach 16 Jahren. Acta oto-lar. *24:* 213–221 (1936).

373 Schmidekam, J.: Experimentelle Studien zur Physiologie des Gehörorgans; Inaug.-Diss., Kiel (1868).

374 Schnurbusch, F.: Über die Bedeutung des Frequenzspektrums von Schallvorgängen bei der Entstehung schalltraumatischer Trommelfellperforationen. Arch. Ohr.-Nas.-KehlkHeilk. *164:* 358–364 (1954).

375 Schönherr, K.H.: Paukenhöhlenfremdkörper beim Schweissen. HNO *4:* 47–49 (1953).

376a Schröer, R.: Zwei traumatische Mittelohrcholesteatome. Z: Laryng. Rhinol. *37:* 573–581 (1958).

376b Schubert, H.: Über die Widerstandsfähigkeit des Trommelfells gegen Überdruck der Aussenluft. HNO *1:* 357–358 (1949).

377 Schuknecht, H.: A clinical study of auditory damage following blows to the head. Ann. Otol., St Louis *59:* 331–358 (1950).

378 Schulthess, G. v.: Facialislähmungen nach Schädelbasisfrakturen. Z. Lar. Rhinol. *40:* 404–409 (1961).

379 Schulthess, G. v.: Tubenfunktionsstörung nach Mittelgesichtsfraktur. Practica oto-rhino-lar. *25:* 393–394 (1963).

380 Schulthess, G. v.; Dubs, R.: Zur Frage der Nervendekompression bei posttraumatischen Facialislähmungen. Practica oto-rhino-lar. *19:* 169–191 (1957).

381 Schulze, E.: Beitrag zur Pathogenese und Klinik des traumatischen Ohrcholesteatoms. HNO *12:* 128–134 (1964).

382 Schwartze, H.: Stichverletzung des Ohres mit Ausfluss von Liquor cerebrospinalis. Arch. Ohrenheilk. *17:* 117–123 (1881).

383 Schwartze, H.: Die chirurgischen Krankheiten des Ohres, Bd 32 (Enke, Stuttgart 1885).

384 Schwartze, H.; Eysell: Über die künstliche Eröffnung des Warzenfortsatzes. Arch. Ohrenheilk. *7:* 157–187 (1873).

385 Schwarz, M.: Die Schleimhäute des Ohres und der Luftwege. Biologie und Klinik (Springer, Berlin 1949).

386 Schwarz, M.: Das Cholesteatom im Gehörgang und im Mittelohr (Thieme, Stuttgart 1966).

387 Schwarz, M.: Topische Diagnose der traumatischen Carotisruptur durch gezielte Gefässzügelung. HNO 6:221 (1956/57).

388 Schwerdtfeger, F.P.; Schwerdtfeger, E.M.: Chirurgische Behandlung der Sofortparese des N. facialis bei Pyramidenlängsfrakturen. Z. Lar. Rhinol. 58:149–153 (1979).

389 Schwetz, F.: Die operative Wiederherstellung der traumatisch unterbrochenen Gehörknöchelchenkette. HNO 24:306–308 (1976).

390 Seaman, R.W.; Newell, R.C.: Another etiology of middle ear cholesteatoma. Archs Otolar. 94:440–442 (1971).

391 Seiferth, L.B.: Ein Beitrag zur Cholesteatomgenese. Traumatisch entstandenes Mittelohr-Cholesteatom. HNO 9:269–271 (1961).

392 Seiferth, L.B.: Über progrediente Schwerhörigkeit nach Detonation und Explosion. Z. Lar. Rhinol. 58:295–302 (1979).

393 Seifi, A.E.: Emergency repair of traumatic drum tears. ORL 38:294–297 (1976).

394 Serbinenko, F.A.: Balloon catheterization and occlusion of major cerebral vessels. J. Neurosurg. 41:125–145 (1974).

395 Shapiro, S.L.: Disarticulation of the incus. Eye Ear Nose Throat Mon. 46:922–927 (1967).

396 Silbiger, H.: Über das Ausmass der Mastoidpneumatisation beim Menschen. Acta anat. 11:215 (1950); cit. Flisberg, K.; et al.: Clinical volume determination of the air-filled ear space. Acta oto-lar. 182: suppl., pp. 39–42 (1963).

397 Silverstein, H.; Fabian, R.L.; Stoll, S.E.; Hong, S.W.: Penetrating wounds of the tympanic membrane and ossicular chain. Trans. Am. Acad. Ophthal. Oto-lar. 77:125–135 (1973).

398 Simmons, F.B.: Theory of membrane breaks in sudden hearing loss. Archs Otolar. 88:41–48 (1968).

399 Simmons, F.B.: The double-membrane break syndrome in sudden hearing loss. Laryngoscope, St Louis 89:59–66 (1979).

400 Simmons, F.B.; Burton, R.D.; Beatty, D.: Round window injury: auditory behavioural and electrophysiological consequences in the cat. Trans. Am. Acad. Ophthal. Oto-lar. 66:715–722 (1962).

401 Simmons, F.B.; Mongeon, C.J.: Endolymphatic duct pressure produces cochlear damage. Archs Otolar. 85:143–150 (1967).

402 Singh, D.; Ahluwalia, K.J.S.: Blast injuries of the ear. J. Laryng. 82:1017–1027 (1968).

403 Singleton, G.T.; Schuknecht, H.F.: Experimental fracture of the stapes in cats. Ann Otol., St Louis 68:1069–1081 (1959).

404 Skolnik, E.M.; Ferrer, J.C.: Cerebrospinal otorrhea. Archs Otolar. 70:795–799 (1959).

405 Skurczynski, W.; Bruchmüller, W.: Facialisschäden bei Schädelbasisfrakturen. Z. ärztl. Fortbild. 70:1168–1170 (1976).

406 Smyth, G.D.L.: Management of ossicular chain defects. J. Laryng. 81:1325–1335 (1967).

407 Sonnenkalb: Die Darstellung des pneumatischen Systems beim Lebenden. Verh. dt. otol. Ges. 22:367–371 (1913).

408 Spector, G.J.; Pettit, W.J.; Davis, G.; Strauss, M.; Rauchbach, E.: Fetal respiratory distress causing CNS and inner ear hemmorhage. Laryngoscope, St Louis 88:764–786 (1978).

409 Spector, G.J.; Pratt, L.L.; Randall, G.: A clinical study of delayed reconstruction in ossicular fractures. Laryngoscope, St Louis 83:837–851 (1973).

410 Spitzer, H.; Ritter, K.: Ein Beitrag zum Tullio-Phänomen. Z. Laryng. Rhinol. *58:*934–936 (1979).

411 Sprem, N.: Les brûlures de l'oreille externe et de la caisse: à propos d'un cas. J. fr. Oto-Rhino-Laryng. *25:* 569–570 (1976).

412 Steinbach, E.: Die Gehörgangsstenose als Folge der fibrösen Dysplasie. Arch. Ohr.-Nas.-KehlkHeilk. *202:*623–627 (1972).

413 Steinbach, E.: Experimental studies on cholesteatoma formation. Acta oto-rhino-lar. belg. *34:*56–61 (1980).

414 Steinmann, K.B.: Ein Wurm im Warzenfortsatz. Mschr. Ohrenheilk. *65:*222–225 (1931).

415 Stenger, P.: Beitrag zur Kenntnis der nach Kopfverletzungen auftretenden Veränderungen im inneren Ohr. Arch. Ohrenheilk. *79:*43–69 (1909).

416 Stenger, P.: Über die chirurgischen und otochirurgischen Indikationen bei der Behandlung von Erkrankungen des Gehörorgans, der Nase und der Nasennebenhöhlen, in besonderer Berücksichtigung kriegschirurgischer Erfahrungen. Beitr. Anat. etc., Ohr *12:*104–118 (1919).

417 Stenger, P.: Zur Diagnostik der Schädelbasisbrüche. Z. Hals-Nasen-Ohrenheilk. *21:*532–538 (1928).

418 Steurer, O.: Traumatische Cholesteatomentstehung. Arch. Ohr.-Nas.-KehlkHeilk. *154:*169–182 (1944).

419 Stewart, T.J.; Belal, A.: Surgical anatomy and pathology of the round window. Clin. Otolaryngol. *6:*45–62 (1981).

420 Strebel, P.: Therapie der traumatischen Trommelfellperforation. HNO *27:*142–144 (1979).

421 Stroud, M.H.; Calcaterra, T.C.: Spontaneous perilymph fistulas. Laryngoscope, St Louis *80:*479–487 (1970).

422 Strupler, W.: Frakturen und Luxationen der Gehörknöchelchen. ORL *25:*53–54 (1963).

423 Sudderth, M.E.: Tympanoplasty in blast-induced perforation. Archs Otolar. *99:*157–159 (1974).

424 Szenes, S.: Über traumatische Läsionen des Gehörorganes. Arch. Ohrenheilk. *43:*58–64 (1897).

425 Tainmont, J.; Uytenhoef: Les anomalies de l'aqueduc cochléaire et leurs conséquences. Acta oto-rhino-lar. belg. *29:*532–539 (1975).

426 Taylor, P.N.; Bicknell, P.G.: Rupture of the round window membrane. Ann. Otol., St Louis *85:* 105–110 (1976).

427 Teodorescu, L.; Stratulat, E.; Cornea, I.; Teodorescu, H.N.: Traumatismele scaritei. (Injuries of the stapes.) Revue Chir. (Otorinolaryngol.) *19:*251–262 (1974).

428 Teodorescu, L.; Stratulat, E.; Cornea, I.: Les traumatismes de la chaîne ossiculaire. Ann. Otolaryngol. Chir. Cervicofac. *92:*319–330 (1975).

429 Terrahe, K.: Die Röntgendiagnostik der Frakturen des Schläfenbeines und der Luxation der Gehörknöchel. Z. Lar. Rhinol. *45:*313–319 (1966).

430 Theuer, J.: Traumaticke poruseni retezu sluchovych kustek a jeho tomograficka diagnostika. (Traumatic damage of the ear ossicles and its tomographic diagnosis.) Čs. Radiol. *27:*252–258 (1973).

431 Thomsen, K.A.: Investigations on the tubal function and measurement of the middle ear pressure in pressure chamber. Acta oto-lar. *140:* suppl., pp. 269–278 (1957).

432a Thorburn, I.B.: Post-traumatic conduction deafness. J. Laryng. *71:*542–545 (1957).

432b Thulin, A.: Traumatic cholesteatoma. Acta oto-lar. *35:*575–582 (1947).

433 Tobeck, A.: Über Trommelfellschädigungen und Hörstörungen nach Detonationen. Arch. Ohr.-Nas.-KehlkHeilk. *150:*41–58 (1941).

434 Tonkin, J.P.; Fagan, P.: Rupture of the round window membrane. J. Laryng. *89:*733–756 (1975).

435 Tonndorf, J.: Verbal communication (1982).

436 Tos, M.: Fractura ossis temporalis. Forlobet og folger af 248 petrosafrakturer. (Fractures of the temporal bone. The courses and sequelae of 248 fractures of the petrous temporal bone.) Ugeskr. Laeg. *133:*1449–1456 (1971).

437 Tos, M.: Prognosis of hearing loss in temporal bone fractures. J. Laryng. *85:*1147–1159 (1971).

438 Tos, M.: Course of and sequelae to 248 petrosal fractures. Acta oto-lar. *75:*353–354 (1973).

439 Tos, M.: Post-traumatic cerebrospinal fluid otorrhoea. ORL *35:*30–35 (1973).

440 Travis, L.W.; Stalnaker, R.L.; Melvin, J.W.: Impact trauma of the human temporal bone. J. Trauma *17:*761–766 (1977).

441 Tyler, T.C.: Pressure trauma to the ears and hearing loss. J. Fla med. Ass. *65:*708–711 (1978).

442 Uffenorde, W.: Histologische Befunde am Felsenbein bei Schädelschussverletzung als Beitrag zur Frage der Kommotionsschwerhörigkeit. Beitr. Anat etc., Ohr *21:*292–324 (1924).

443 Ulrich, K.: Verletzungen des Gehörorgans bei Schädelbasisfrakturen. Acta oto-lar. *6:* suppl., pp. 1–150 (1926).

444 Van den Eeckhaut, J.: Pathogénie et évolution des fractures ossiculaires. Bases expérimentales et cliniques. Acta oto-rhino-lar. belg. *23:*33–54 (1969).

445 Venker, J.: The missing incus. ORL *35:*237–240 (1973).

446 Vick, U.: Verbrennungen des Mittelohres durch Schweissperlen. Z. ärztl. Fortbild. *72:*726–728 (1978).

447 Vignaud, J.; Sultan. A.: Dislocations traumatiques de la chaîne des osselets. J. belge Radiol. *54:*203–208 (1971).

448 Vilar-Puig, P.; Fernandes, A.; Lopez, F.: Hipoacusia conductiva en el traumatizado de craneo. Presentación de dos casos. Acta oto-rino-laring. ibero-amer. *19:*201–208 (1968).

449 Voss, O.: Operatives Vorgehen bei Schädelbasisfrakturen bei Mitbeteiligung von Ohr und Nase. Beitr. Anat. etc., Ohr *3:*385–405 (1910).

450 Voss, O.: Die Chirurgie der Schädelbasisfrakturen auf Grund 25-jähriger Erfahrungen (Barth, Leipzig 1936).

451 Wagenhäuser, G.J.: Bericht über die Universitätspoliklinik für Ohrenkranke zu Tübingen. Arch. Ohrenheilk. *27:*156–174 (1889).

452 Wahl, E. v.: Über Fracturen der Schädelbasis; in Volkmann, Sammlung klinischer Vorträge. *228:*1945–1970 (1883).

453 Walb, H.: Krankheiten der Paukenhöhle und der Tuba Eustachii; in Schwartze, Handbuch der Ohrenheilkunde, Bd II, pp. 186–298 (Vogel, Leipzig 1893).

454 Waltner, J.G.: Barrier membrane of the cochlear aqueduct. Histologic studies on the patency of the cochlear aqueduct. Archs Otolar. *47:*656–669 (1948).

455 Waltner, J.G.; Weissman, B.; Kovar, M.: Healing of stapedial fractures in humans. Laryngoscope, St Louis *81:*962–970 (1971).

456 Weber, M.: Über den regelwidrigen Röntgenbefund bei chronischer Mittelohreiterung. Z. Hals-Nasen-Ohrenheilk. *48:*465–477 (1943).

457 Wederstrandt: Verbrennung durch Eingiessen von geschmolzenem Blei. Am. J. med.

Sci. (1852); cit. Passow, A.: Die Verletzung des Gehörorganes (Bergmann, Wiesbaden 1905).

458 Wehmer: Über Verletzung des Ohres vom gerichtsärztlichen Standpunkt. Friedreichs Blätter gerichtl. Med. *36:*37 (1885/86); cit. Imhofer, R.: Gerichtliche Ohrenheilkunde (Kabitzsch, Leipzig 1920).

459 Weilepp, M.; Rentzsch, G.: Ergebnisse der konservativen Tympanoplastik bei traumatischen Trommelfellperforationen. HNO *18:*245–248 (1970).

460 Weisskopf, A.; Murphy, J.T.; Merzenich, M.M.: Genesis of the round window rupture syndrome; some experimental observations. Laryngoscope, St Louis *88:*389–397 (1978).

461 Wicke, W.: Die Bedeutung der Pneumatisation für den Frakturverlauf und die Entstehung von Facialisparesen bei Schläfenbeinbrüchen. Mschr. Ohrenheilk. *108:*425–428 (1974).

462 Williams, D.J.; Simpson, D.A.; Savage, J.P.: Cerebrospinal fluid otorhinorrhoea investigation and management. J. Laryng. *91:*433–434 (1977).

463 Williams, R.A.: Head injury with fracture of stapes. J. Laryng. *72:*666–670 (1958).

464 Willis, R.: Tympanotomy. 2. Traumatic middle ear lesions. J. Otolaryngol. Soc. Aust. *3:*47–50 (1970).

465 Winckler, G.: Observations concernant l'aqueduc du limaçon. ORL *25:*50–52 (1963).

466 Wittmaack, K.: Kritische Bemerkungen zu der Arbeit 'Das Mittelohr-Cholesteatom' von Privatdozent Dr. J. Berberich. Beitr. Anat. etc., Ohr *27:*1–5 (1929).

467 Wittmaack, K.: Über die traumatische Labyrinthdegeneration. Arch. Ohr.-Nas.-KehlkHeilk. *131:* 59–124 (1932).

468 Wlodyka, J.: Studies on cochlear aqueduct patency. Ann. Otol., St Louis *87:*22–28 (1978).

469 Wodak, E.: Zum Mittelohrcholesteatom traumatischer Genese. Z. Lar. Rhinol. *41:*117–120 (1962).

470 Wolff, D.; Bellucci, R.J.: The human ossicular ligaments. Ann. Otol., St Louis 65:895–910 (1956).

471 Wullstein, H.L.: Die Methode der Dekompression des N. facialis vom Austritt aus dem Labyrinth bis zum Foramen stylomastoideum ohne Beeinträchtigung des Mittelohres. Arch. Ohr.-Nas.-KehlkHeilk. *172:*582–587 (1958).

472 Yanagisawa, E.; Shimada, T.; Hughes, M.: Fractures of the stapes. Report of a case. Conn. Med. *37:*565–567 (1973).

473 Zalewski, T.: Experimentelle Untersuchungen über die Resistenzfähigkeit des Trommelfells. Z. Ohrenheilk. *52:*109–128 (1906).

474 Zangemeister: Die Hamburger Erfahrungen bei Luftstossschäden des Ohres. HNO *1:*136–137 (1948).

475 Zaufal, E.: Casuistische Beiträge zu den traumatischen Verletzungen des Trommelfelles. Teil I. Arch. Ohrenheilk. *7:* 188–205 (1873).

476 Zaufal, E.: Casuistische Beiträge zu den traumatischen Verletzungen des Trommelfelles. Teil II. Arch. Ohrenheilk. *7:* 280–287 (1873).

477 Zaufal, E.: Casuistische Beiräge zu den traumatischen Verletzungen des Trommelfells. Tel III. Arch. Ohrenheilk. *8:* 31–49 (1874).

478 Ziv, M.; Philipsohn, N.C.; Leventon, G.; Man, A.: Blast injury of the ear: treatment and evaluation. Milit. Med. *138:* 811–813 (1973).

479 Zöllner, F.: Widerstandsmessungen an der Ohrtrompete. Arch. Ohr.-Nas.-KehlkHeilk. *140:* 137–154 (1936).

480 Zonis, R.D.: Eardrum perforation. Med. Trial. Tech. Q. *18:* 31–34 (1971).

Part B

This part lists a number of references that were added at the time of final editing. Their order numbers are continuous with those of part A.

481 Bárány, E.: A contribution to the physiology of bone conduction. Acta oto-lar. *26:* suppl., pp. 1–223 (1938).

482 Dancer, A.L.; Franke, A.B.; Smigielski, P.; Albe, F.; Fogot, H.: Holographic interferometry applied to the investigation of tympanic-membrane displacements in guinea pig ears subjected to acoustic impulses. J. Acoust. Soc. Am. *58:* 223–228 (1975).

483 Fletcher, H.: Speech and hearing (Van Nostrand, New York 1929).

484 Goodhill, V.: Ear diseases, deafness and dizziness (Harper & Row, Hagerstown 1979).

485 Graham, M.: Personal communication (1982).

486 Helmholtz, H.: Die Mechanik der Gehörknöchelchen und des Trommelfells. Pflüger's Arch. ges. Physiol. *1:* 1–60 (1868); Translated as: The mechanism of the ossicles of the ear and the membrana tympani (Woods, New York 1873).

487 Khanna, S.M.; Tonndorf, J.: The vibratory pattern of the round window in cats. J. Acoust. Soc. Am. *50:* 1474–1483 (1972).

488 Khanna, S.M.; Tonndorf, J.: Tympanic membrane vibrations in cats, studied by time-averaged holography. J. Acoust. Soc. Am. *51:* 1904–1920 (1972).

489 Kobrak, H.: Construction material of the sound conducting system of the human ear. J. Acoust. Soc. Am. *20:* 125–130 (1948).

490 Kruger, B.; Tonndorf, J.: Middle-ear transmission in cats with experimentally induced tympanic membrane perforations. J. Acoust. Soc. Am. *61:* 126–132 (1977).

491 Lawrence, M.; Yantis, P.A.: Onset and growth of aural harmonics in the overloaded ear. J. Acoust. Soc. Am. *28:* 852–858 (1956).

492 Rieker, E.O.: Tierexperimentelle Untersuchung der Veränderungen des Ohres nach Luftdruckschwankungen. Arch. Ohr.-Nas.-KehlkHeilk. *155:* 194–205 (1948).

493 Tjernström, O.; Casselbrandt, M.: Pressure chamber treatment in acute attacks of Menière's disease; in Vosteen, Schuknecht, Pfaltz, et al., Menière's disease, p. 211 (Thieme, Stuttgart 1981).

494 Tonndorf, J.: The influence of service in submarines on the auditory organ. D-2 in German Submarine Medicine in WW II (US Navy, 1948).

495 Tonndorf, J.; Baker, D.C.; Bernstein, L.; Campbell, R.A.; Cottle, R.D.; Duvall, A.J.; Greenfield, E.C.; Kaufman, R.S.; King, A.F.; Olesen, M.; Reneau, J.P.; Voots, R.J.: Bone conduction. Acta oto-lar. *213:* Suppl., pp. 1–123 (1966).

496 Tonndorf, J.; Khanna, S.M.: Some properties of sound transmission in the middle and outer ears of cats. J. Acoust. Soc. Am. *41:* 513–521 (1967).

497 Tonndorf, J.; Khanna, S.M.: Tympanic membrane vibrations in human cadaver ears, studied by time-averaged holography. J. Acoust. Soc. Am. *52:* 1221–1233 (1972).

498 Voldrich, L.: Mechanical properties of basilar membrane. Acta oto-lar. *86:* 331–335 (1978).

499 Wiener, F.M.; Ross, D.A.: Pressure distribution in the auditory canal in a progressive sound field. J. Acoust. Soc. Am. *18:* 401–408 (1946).

500 Zwislocki, J.J.: Some measurements of impedance at the eardrum. J. Acoust. Soc. Am. *29:* 349–356 (1957).

501 Zwislocki, J.J.: Some impedance measurements in normal and pathological ears. J. Acoust. Soc. Am. *29:* 1312–1317 (1957).

502 Zwislocki, J.J.; Feldman, A.S.: Post-mortem acoustic impedance of human ears. J. Acoust. Soc. Am. *35:* 104–107 (1963).

Subject Index